Management of the Patient in Labor

Management of the Patient in Labor

MORTON A. STENCHEVER, M.D.
Professor and Chairman
Department of Obstetrics and Gynecology
University of Washington School of Medicine
Seattle, Washington

TANYA SORENSEN, M.D.
Clinical Assistant Professor
Division of Maternal and Fetal Medicine
Department of Obstetrics and Gynecology
University of Washington School of Medicine
Seattle, Washington

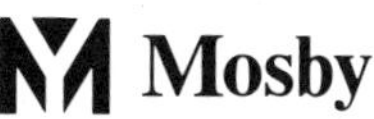

St. Louis Baltimore Boston Chicago London Philadelphia Sydney Toronto

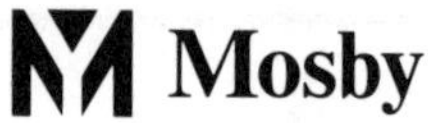

Dedicated to Publishing Excellence

Sponsoring Editor: Stephanie Manning
Developmental Editor: Laura DeYoung
Associate Managing Editor, Manuscript Services: Deborah Thorp
Production Manager: Nancy C. Baker
Proofroom Manager: Barbara M. Kelly

A C.V. Mosby imprint of Mosby-Year Book, Inc.

Mosby-Year Book, Inc., 11830 Westline Industrial Drive, St. Louis, MO 63146

2 3 4 5 6 7 8 9 0 CL/MA 97 96 95 94 93

Library of Congress Cataloging-in-Publication Data
Stenchever, Morton A.
Management of the patient in labor / Morton A. Stenchever, Tanya Sorensen.
p. cm.
Includes bibliographical references and index.
ISBN 0801676355
1. Labor (Obstetrics) 2. Labor (Obstetrics)—Complications.
I. Sorensen, Tanya. II. Title.
[DNLM: 1. Delivery. 2. Labor. WQ 300 S825m 1993]
RG651.S74 1993 92-48352
618.4—dc20 CIP
DNLM/DLC
for Library of Congress

PREFACE

This manual is written specifically for the medical student, intern, or nurse practitioner who is experiencing his/her first encounter with laboring patients. It outlines the physiological, psychological, and physical factors that influence the progress of labor, demonstrates the tools available for monitoring the progress of a laboring patient, and offers suggestions for managing problems that may arise. The approaches used are practical and should help the learner obtain the maximum educational experience while following a patient throughout labor and delivery. Since very little replaces practical experience, the learner is urged to remain at the bedside of the patient throughout labor so that the precepts defined in this manual can be directly observed and understood in the clinical setting.

Morton A. Stenchever, M.D.
Tanya Sorensen, M.D.

CONTENTS

INTRODUCTION: THE IMPORTANCE OF PRENATAL CARE

1

The public health benefits of prenatal care are well documented; regular prenatal care can substantially reduce maternal and perinatal morbidity and mortality. Adequate prenatal care can also reduce the risks and uncertainties of labor management. Unfortunately, such care is often most important for patients who find it least available. The care giver confronted with a patient in labor must be skilled in rapid ascertainment of risk by history and physical examination.

Optimal women's health care includes preconceptional counseling. For women with chronic illness such as hypertension or diabetes mellitus, counseling is used to make patients aware of the need and means for optimal disease control prior to pregnancy. For example, the diabetic may be at risk for fetal anomalies, uteroplacental insufficiency, or macrosomia and shoulder dystocia. These risks may be reduced with glycemic control. Information on nutrition, genetic risks, and teratogens are also dispersed at the preconceptual visit. Risks of birth defects due to hyperglycemia, drug use, or environmental exposure are highest during embryogenesis; some defects occur before the patient is even aware of her pregnancy. Behavior modification as the patient is attempting to conceive is thus essential. Finally, particularly in the patient at medical or genetic risk, early identification of pregnancy and prompt prenatal care will ensure the availability of services and options for optimal pregnancy outcome.

Patient education must continue throughout the preconceptual, prenatal, puerperal, and postpartum periods. The concern of a mother for her child is remarkable, and most patients are very receptive to information that will improve pregnancy outcome. Pregnancy is also a good time to provide parenting education; care of a newborn infant is extremely stressful and seldom what the new mother expects. Constant communication builds knowledge and confidence and greatly improves the pregnancy and delivery experience. A list of topics to be discussed during prenatal visits is presented in Table 1–1.

Following the diagnosis of pregnancy, the first prenatal visit should occur during the first trimester. The focus of this visit, as for most prenatal care, is identification of risk. A comprehensive history is essential. Information concerning the current pregnancy should include symptoms such as nausea, bleeding, urinary symptoms, and fevers or rashes. A thorough menstrual history is necessary, and the gynecologic history should also include a history of sexually transmitted diseases. A maternal medical his-

TABLE 1–1.
Ongoing Education at Prenatal Visits

First trimester
Nutrition
Seat belts
Sexuality
Warning signs
Substance use/environmental exposures
Second trimester
Exercise
Prenatal classes
Fetal movement
Warning signs
Third trimester
Preparation for labor delivery
Warning signs
Discomforts of late pregnancy
Postpartum issues including breast-feeding
Birth plan

tory with particular attention to chronic illness and medication use should be obtained. A surgical history with attention to pelvic and abdominal operations and blood transfusions is also important. Features of previous pregnancies can be very helpful in ascertaining risk. A prior history of cephalopelvic disproportion, for example, may alert the clinician to pay close attention to pelvic type and progress in labor. Genetic risk factors include maternal and paternal age and family history of birth defects. Finally, the social history should include substance use, nutrition, and life-style factors and stresses.

Physical examination at the first prenatal visit must be comprehensive. Often the pregnant patient will not have had a thorough physical examination since early childhood. Abnormalities of the general physical examination such as elevated blood pressure or a heart murmur require further workup. Uterine and pelvic size and shape are also ascertained. Determination of uterine size along with menstrual history is used to date the pregnancy; accurate dating may become important in management decisions at the time of labor. Again, abnormalities or inconsistencies on physical examination call for directed laboratory examination.

Laboratory data are collected routinely at the first prenatal visit; again, the focus is risk identification (Table 1–2). Blood type and Rh factor along with an indirect Coombs' test are obtained. Other tests include hematocrit, hepatitis antigen, rubella antibody, urine culture, syphilis serology, and Papanicolaou smear. In patients with risk factors, gonorrhea and chlamydia cultures and human immunodeficiency virus serologies are obtained. If pregnancy dating or viability are in question or if multiple pregnancy or fetal anomalies are suspected, ultrasound is offered. As mentioned above, abnormalities noted by history or on physical examination may require directed laboratory follow-up.

It is worth noting here that pregnancy, labor, and delivery involve extreme physiologic changes. Patients with well-compensated or even undetected illness may become quite

TABLE 1–2.
Routine Laboratory Tests in Pregnancy

All Pregnancies	At-Risk Pregnancies Only
First visit	
Blood type—Rh/indirect Coombs' test	Gonorrhea cervical culture
Hematocrit	Chlamydial cervical culture
Hepatitis antigen	Human immunodeficiency virus serology
Rubella antibody	
Urine culture	
Syphilis serology	
Papanicolaou smear	
16–20 weeks' visit	
Pregnancy risk profile or maternal serum α-fetoprotein	Screening ultrasound
26–28 weeks' visit	
Glucose	Repeat indirect Coombs'
Repeat hematocrit	Repeat sexually transmitted disease screen

ill with the stress of pregnancy or labor. For example, cardiac output and heart rate increase markedly by the late first trimester; in labor the cardiovascular load increases further with the autotransfusion caused by each uterine contraction and the tachycardia caused by pain. Postpartum, tremendous mobilization of extravascular fluid to the intravascular space occurs. Such changes, while easily tolerated by healthy women, may cause pulmonary edema or cardiovascular collapse in the previously well compensated cardiac patient. Other examples of unmasking of disease during pregnancy in apparently healthy patients include those with renal disease or hypertension. In these patients, careful evaluation to identify previously unknown illness is essential.

Prenatal visits subsequent to the first are scheduled at regular intervals (Table 1–3). In first and second trimesters, monthly visits are adequate in uncomplicated pregnancies. After 28 weeks, the frequency of visits should increase to biweekly, and in the last month of pregnancy, weekly visits are appropriate. Milestones in early pregnancy that should be recorded include identification of fetal heart tones by Doppler ultrasound at 12 weeks and by fetoscope at 20 weeks and the onset of perceptible fetal movement at 16 to 22 weeks. When indicated, genetic counseling should be offered early in pregnancy to allow the use of chorionic villous sampling at 9 to 11 weeks or amniocentesis at 16 to 20 weeks. A maternal serum α-fetoprotein or pregnancy risk profile (α-fetoprotein, estriol, and human

TABLE 1–3.
Frequency of Visits During Pregnancy*

Trimester	Frequency
1st	Monthly
2nd	Monthly
3rd	2-wk intervals to 36 wk, then weekly

*Primigravida with uncomplicated pregnancy.

chorionic gonadotropin) should be offered at 16 to 20 weeks. These blood tests can identify women at risk for neural tube defects (increased α-fetoprotein concentration) or Down syndrome (decreased α-fetoprotein, decreased estriol, and increased human chorionic gonadotropin levels). Definitive testing by amniocentesis can then be offered. A 50-g 1-hour glucose challenge is performed at 28 weeks along with a repeat hematocrit. In Rh-negative patients, a repeat indirect Coombs' test is performed at the same time and, if negative, Rh_o (D) immune globulin (Rhogam) given to prevent sensitization to the Rh antigen. A repeat infection screen (human immunodeficiency virus, hepatitis antigen, gonorrhea, *Chlamydia,* syphilis serology) is also indicated in high-risk patients at 28 weeks. High-risk patients with a negative hepatitis screen should be immunized after their first prenatal visit.

Third trimester visits focus on maternal blood pressure and weight gain as well as fetal (fundal) growth. Education continues to be important, and all patients should be made aware of warning signs such as bleeding, pain, swelling, and headache (Table 1–4). Significant bleeding in late pregnancy is almost always ominous and requires immediate evaluation for placental abruption, premature labor, placenta previa, or vasa previa. Approximately 7% of primigravid patients develop preeclampsia, a condition that may be life-threatening for mother and baby. Prompt recognition can prevent adverse outcomes in most cases. Progressive fetal growth and active fetal movement are normal in pregnancy; the absence of either or excessive

TABLE 1–4.
Symptoms and Signs of Preeclampsia

Symptoms
Swelling
Headache
Scotoma
Epigastric pain
Vaginal bleeding
Decreased fetal movement
Signs
Elevated blood pressure (≥15 points diastolic or ≥30 points systolic over first-trimester levels)
Rapid weight gain (≥5 lb in 1 wk)
Edema
Proteinuria (≥1+ on dipstick of urine)

uterine growth should alert the clinician to the need for fetal surveillance with heart rate testing or ultrasound evaluation. Such testing is also indicated in pregnancies complicated by known maternal or fetal disease.

The third trimester is the time to encourage attendance at prenatal classes. These can be an important adjunct to the clinician's ongoing patient education. In particular, a detailed review of labor and delivery prepares the patient for an otherwise potentially overwhelming experience. Nonpharmacologic pain control methods are taught in many prenatal classes and can reduce the need for anesthetic by as much as 30%.

When a patient who has had no prenatal care presents in labor, risk factors must be rapidly identified. A focused history, physical examination, and laboratory assessment must be obtained. Maternal symptoms and medical, surgical, and social histories are quickly reviewed. An examination directed to vital signs, heart, lungs, abdomen, and pelvis is performed. Gestational age and the condition of the fetus are determined, often with the aid of ultrasound. Screening laboratory tests usually obtained at the first prenatal visit are collected; other laboratory tests such as the pregnancy risk profile, genetic studies, and glucose screening are forgone. Emotional support, reassurance, and education must be supplied to the extent possible.

Pregnancy is as varied as people, and this summary is not intended as a comprehensive guide to prenatal care. Rather, we point out that labor occurs as part of a continuum that begins before conception. Identification of pregnancy risk factors and appropriate therapy for identified abnormalities can allow optimal success and minimal complications in labor.

ADDITIONAL READING

American Academy of Pediatrics/American College of Obstetricians and Gynecologists: *Guidelines for Perinatal Care*. American Academy of Pediatrics, Washington, DC, 1991.

Hobel CJ, Hyrarinen MA, et al: Prenatal and antepartum high risk screening. Prediction of the high risk neonate. *Am J Obstet Gynecol* 1973; 117:1.

FACTORS IN LABOR 2

An interrelationship of factors affect the way in which a woman will labor and whether or not she will have a successful outcome involving vaginal delivery of a healthy child. Seven factors influence the conduct of normal labor:

1. The patient's general physical and emotional condition
2. The size of the fetus
3. The presentation of the fetus
4. The quality and type of uterine contractions
5. The condition of the cervix
6. Uterine anatomy and volume
7. Architecture of the bony pelvis

Each of these factors will influence labor and must be considered both individually and in an interrelated fashion as the physician manages the conduct of labor.

PATIENT'S GENERAL PHYSICAL AND EMOTIONAL CONDITION

If the physician has been caring for the patient throughout pregnancy, he/she will have had the opportunity to assess the patient's general health and emotional status. Thus medical conditions that can be corrected will have been dealt with. The patient's nutritional status will have been assessed and, where necessary, improved, and the physician will have had the opportunity to begin to prepare the patient for labor by discussing what will occur at the time of labor and what options with respect to anesthesia, analgesia, and what means of coping are available. The patient and her significant other will have had the opportunity to attend prenatal classes that will have addressed the mechanics of labor and coping mechanisms. Because of these factors the patient ideally will enter labor in a state of good physical and emotional health and with a positive attitude toward the experience.

In a situation where the patient has had little or no antepartum care and is admitted in labor unprepared and unevaluated, the physician will have to rapidly assess her physical and emotional status and establish a plan for management that takes her status into consideration.

Most patients who are admitted in labor are screened for infectious disease states such as herpes virus and group B streptococcal colonization. Usually an intravenous catheter is inserted and blood for hematocrit determination and for storage in case a crossmatch is necessary is drawn. The urine is checked for the presence of protein, and the patient is given a short physical examination that addresses the state of her hydration and her blood pressure, temperature, and pulse. An evaluation of her heart and breath sounds is made by auscultation, and her abdomen is examined to derive information with respect to fetal size and position and fetal heart rate. If there is no excessive vaginal bleeding, the patient usually undergoes a vaginal examination to assess the condition of the membranes and the dilatation and the effacement of the cervix. The presenting part is identified vaginally if possible and its station noted. These findings will be further discussed later. The presence of ruptured membranes may be noted by fluid coming from the cervix that will "fern" on a microscope slide. Since the pH of amniotic fluid is alkaline, it will turn litmus paper blue or pH paper alkaline.

The presence and quality of the patient's contractions can be noted and also discussed from a historical standpoint. The patient should be asked when her labor started, how often her contractions are coming, and roughly how long they last.

At this point it is appropriate to rediscuss the patient's plans for analgesia and anesthesia and to determine whether or not she plans to breast-feed.

If the patient seems dehydrated, she may be hydrated with intravenous fluids—generally Ringer's lactate solution.

Her questions should be answered in a kind and nonthreatening manner by both physicians and nurses. Examination should be performed gently in order to create as little anxiety as possible. An anxious patient may have elevated serotonin levels that may influence the quality and efficiency of uterine contractions; thus it is important to reduce the patient's anxieties as much as possible.

SIZE OF THE FETUS

The size of the fetus can only be estimated. Even in the most experienced of hands it is difficult to judge the fetal weight by abdominal examination more closely than ±0.5 lb. Ultrasound measurements are available and do improve the accuracy in many instances, but they too will frequently be in considerable error. Successful outcome of labor, that is, appropriate progress of labor and the delivery itself, will be affected by the size of the fetus. The size of the fetus is only half the equation, however; the other is the size of the bony pelvis. A large fetus may be delivered easily through a large pelvis, and a small fetus may be delivered easily through a smaller pelvis. Thus success or failure may be determined by the interrelationship of these two factors.

The art of estimating fetal weight improves with practice; therefore, it is important to try to guess the fetal weight of each patient. A number of factors will influence this estimate. These include the size and weight of the mother, which may be important because a thick abdominal wall in an obese woman will make the fetus appear larger since it is palpated through a thicker body wall. Also, obesity in the mother may make for a larger baby, whereas a woman who is underweight and has not gained much weight will usually have a smaller baby.

The second factor influencing the estimation of fetal weight is parity. As a general rule, babies tend to get larger as the parity increases. Thus if a previous baby weighed 8 lb, it is reasonable to assume that the current child, if at term, will probably weigh at least that much. Clearly there are variations to this rule, but there is a general tendency for fetuses to become larger with increasing parity.

The third factor is the condition of the mother. Diabetic mothers whose condition is not well controlled tend to have larger babies. Mothers who suffer from chronic hypertension or renal disease may have smaller babies.

In general, the normal range of weight for mature babies at term should be between 2500 and 4000 g. Fetuses of pregnancies that are less than term, of course, will be smaller, and fetuses of postmature pregnancies may be larger. Fetuses over 4500 g are in jeopardy for shoulder dystocia should they be delivered vaginally, and physicians must be prepared for this eventuality in such cases. This will be discussed later.

PRESENTATION OF THE FETUS

The most common presentation of the fetus is vertex, or "head first." To describe the position of the presenting vertex the occiput is utilized as a reference point. To locate the occiput during vaginal examination the posterior fontanelle is palpated. It is formed by the junction of the parietal bones and the occipital bone. The most common position in vertex presentations is occipitoanterior, with the head flexed and the face of the fetus toward the mother's back. This allows for the shortest anteroposterior diameter of the fetal skull to be directed through the pelvis and results in efficient progress in descent. Left occipitoanterior (LOA) implies that the occiput is in the maternal left anterior quadrant, and right occipitoanterior (ROA) implies the maternal right anterior quadrant (Fig 2–1).

Degrees of deflection, or "deflection attitudes," of the vertex presentation are observed during labor and may profoundly affect the normal conduct of labor. In the occipitoposterior position the fetal force is toward the pubic symphysis, and poor flexion of the vertex occurs. This requires a longer diameter of the fetal skull to be conducted through the pelvis, thereby reducing the efficiency of the labor.

Extreme examples of deflection are the brow and face presentations (Fig 2–2). In the presence of either, vaginal delivery may be difficult or impossible if the fetus is of normal birth weight. However, during descent and prior to expulsion, a large majority of fetuses in an extreme deflection attitude convert or rotate to a more favorable vertex presentation, thus allowing delivery through the birth canal.

Fetuses with breech presentations are found in approximately 3% to 6% of all deliveries. Vaginal examination utilizes the fetal sacrum as the positional reference point, entirely analogous to the occiput in vertex presentations. The description of the breech presentation, the conduct of labor, and the mode of delivery will vary according to the attitude of the fetal lower extremities. A frank breech pre-

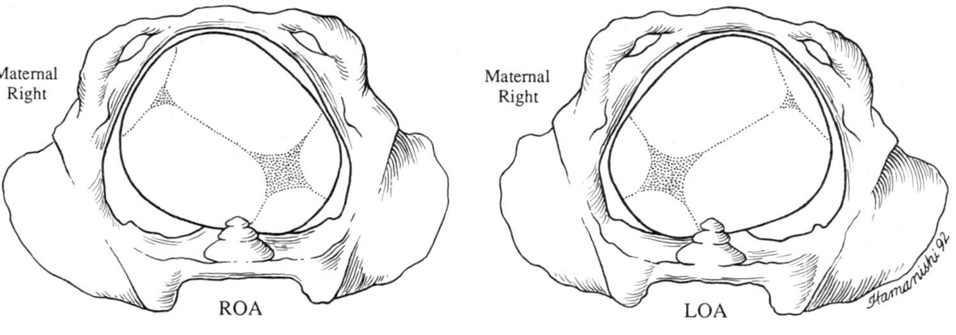

FIG 2–1.
Various positions of the vertex are depicted (ROA and LOA).

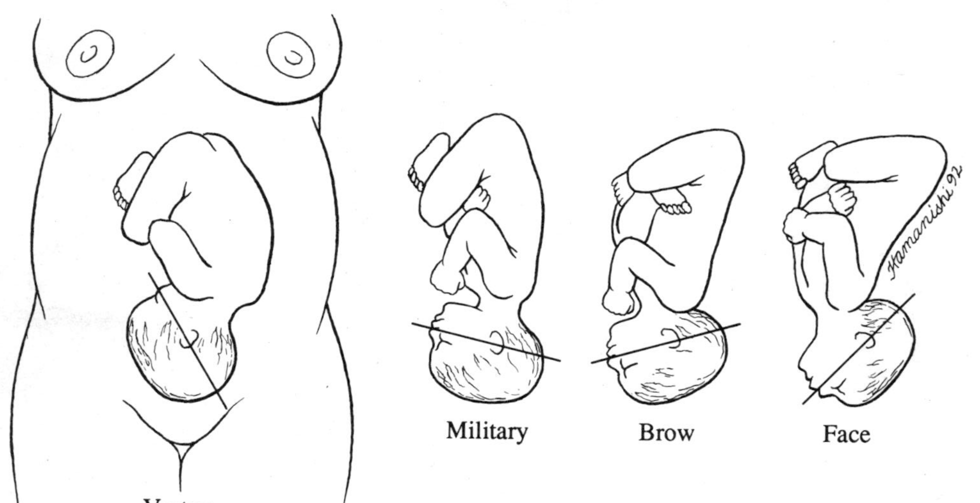

FIG 2–2.
Attitudes of the fetal skull (flexed, military, brow, and face) are depicted.

sentation, that is, one in which the buttocks are presenting but the legs are extended, can usually be managed as a vaginal delivery if the pelvis is deemed adequate. Footling or double-footling breech presentations or complete breech presentations (both feet and buttocks presenting) are customarily delivered by cesarean section (Fig 2–3). The decision of whether or not to deliver a fetus in a breech position vaginally is now a complex issue involving the skill of the obstetrician, the size of the pelvis, the condition of the fetus, and the medicolegal climate that prevails in the community.

Other unusual presentations having a profound effect on the mechanism of normal labor include transverse lie, shoulder presentation, and oblique lie. The management of these require careful evaluation and often cesarean delivery.

QUALITY AND TYPE OF UTERINE CONTRACTIONS

The fourth factor affecting the conduct of normal labor is the force of the uterine contractions. The force of contractions is least in the early first stage of labor, but it increases as progress occurs and dilatation and descent take place. The force of uterine contractions can be directly related to the patient's general condition. Since uterine muscle is no different from any other body tissue with respect to its metabolism, it performs more efficiently when the patient is in optimum metabolic homeostasis. Thus a dehydrated or exhausted patient cannot be expected to have ef-

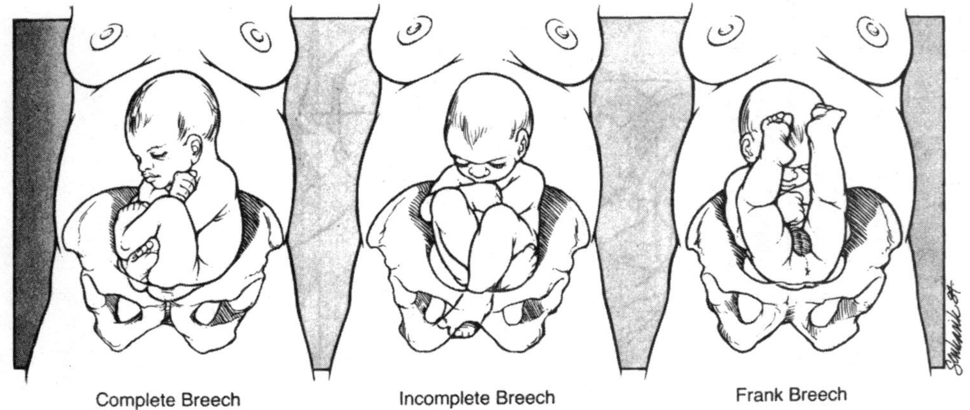

FIG 2–3.
Frank, complete, and incomplete (footling) breech presentations are depicted. (From Gabbe SG, Niebyl JR, Simpson JL: *Obstetrics*. New York, Churchill Livingstone, 1986. Used by permission.)

ficient contractions, and in such cases it may be necessary to rest and hydrate the patient before attempting to improve the quality of contractions.

The quality and force (efficiency) of uterine contractions become compromised in the presence of relative or absolute cephalopelvic disproportion. In such patients, progress in labor may not occur. Arrest in the progress of labor associated with and manifested by changes in the uterine contraction pattern is inertia.

In "hypotonic" uterine inertia, the force of contraction lessens, the interval between contractions lengthens, and neither descent nor dilatation occurs. Therapy in this situation usually includes oxytocin and may be aided by amniotomy, depending on the clinical situation. "Hypertonic" uterine inertia occurs less commonly. In such cases, contractions are tumultuous, shortened in interval, and not coordinated. Therefore, by definition, they are not effective contractions. Tocolytic agents or heavy sedation may be necessary in such a situation.

Efficient uterine contractions are generally present when the strength of the contractions varies between 50 and 100 mm Hg (Fig 2–4). It is possible to measure the strength of contractions by using an internal pressure catheter if the membranes are ruptured or by placing a pressure catheter within the uterine musculature either transvaginally or transabdominally. A spring-gauge tocodynometer such as is found in external fetal monitoring equipment can only estimate the strength of contractions and cannot give an

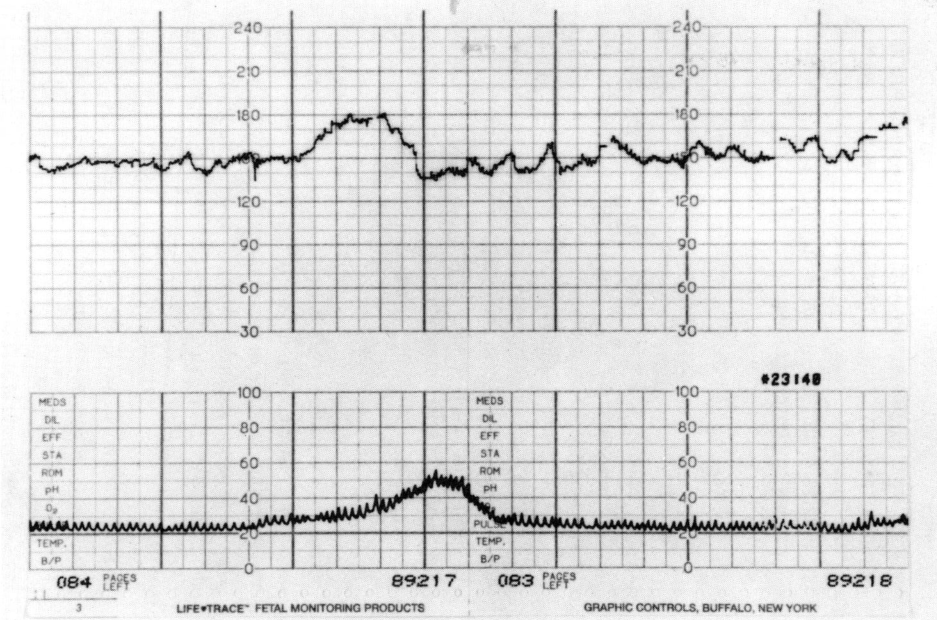
240
210
180
150
120
90
60
30
100
80
60
40
20
0
MEDS
DIL
EFF
STA
ROM
pH
O_2
PULSE
TEMP.
B/P
084 PAGES LEFT
89217
083 PAGES LEFT
89218
#23148
3
LIFE•TRACE™ FETAL MONITORING PRODUCTS
GRAPHIC CONTROLS, BUFFALO, NEW YORK

accurate measurement. It is worthwhile knowing the strength of contractions if oxytocin is to be used in order to determine whether or not an adequate trial of labor is being given and to detect whether the uterus is being hyperstimulated.

CONDITION OF THE CERVIX

The fifth factor is the condition of the cervix. In early labor the cervix may be thick and uneffaced. As labor progresses and uterine muscular activity increases, the cervix becomes softened and flattened, and the lower uterine segment develops. When the substance of the cervix is completely taken up into the lower uterine segment and no longer has any thickness, the cervix is said to be 100% or completely effaced. The effacement is estimated during labor in percentages of complete effacement. Since an uneffaced cervix is roughly 2 cm in length, a 50% effaced cervix is one that is approximately 1 cm in length (Fig 2–5). The physician should not expect efficient labor until effacement has occurred. Primigravidas will frequently efface the cervix during the last 3 weeks of pregnancy and enter labor with a completely effaced cervix. However, if labor is begun in a primigravida with a poorly effaced cervix, a prolonged latent phase can be expected. Multiparas, on the other hand, will frequently soften their cervices without complete effacement prior to labor and may be

---

FIG 2–4.
Internal pressure catheter–generated uterine contraction strip showing a normal contraction pattern (50 to 100 mm Hg).

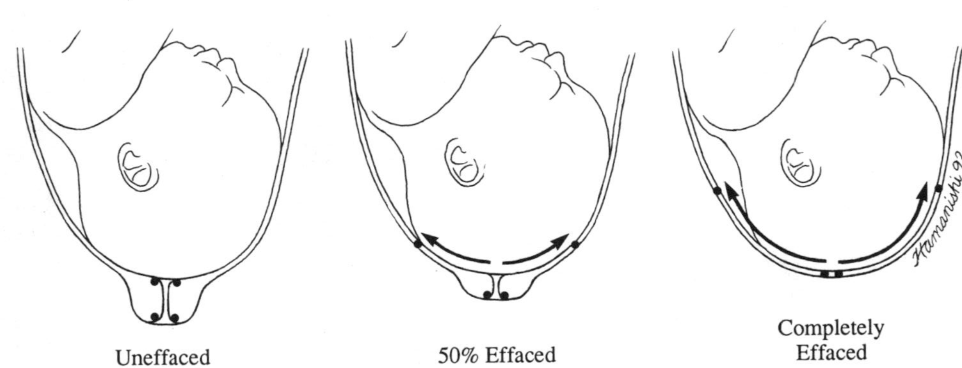

FIG 2–5.
Effacement of the cervix is shown. *Dots* denote the position of the internal and external cervical as labor progresses.

partly dilated even without an effaced cervix. Also, multiparous patients entering labor with a soft cervix that is not well effaced may still dilate and rapidly efface at the same time.

Some labors demonstrate a long period of effacement (latent period), and uterine contractions will be of poor quality and irregular during this time. However, progress in effacement is extremely variable, and the physician must not assume a pathologic condition if this aspect of normal labor does not follow a classic pattern.

Many studies have demonstrated that the condition of the cervix is related to "labor readiness." The degree of dilatation, consistency of the cervix, or both are the most important factors in considering a patient for induction of labor. Thus a patient with a soft, well-effaced cervix and 1 to 3 cm of dilatation can be expected to be inducible with relative ease, whereas an individual with a thick, firm, and undilated cervix can be expected to be resistant to induction. The success of labor induction can be estimated by using information relating to cervical dilation, length, consistency, and position, as well as the station of the head. Table 2–1 outlines how the modified Bishop score is obtained. Roughly 80% of patients with scores of 4 or more can be expected to undergo successful oxytocin induction of labor.

UTERINE ANATOMY AND VOLUME

The sixth factor in labor involves abnormalities in uterine distension and consequent abnormalities in the efficiency

TABLE 2–1.
Modified Bishop Score

	Score			
Parameter	0	1	2	3
Station of the head	3	−2	−1−0	+1−+2
Cervix				
Dilation (cm)	0	1−2	3−4	>4
Length (cm)	3	2	1	0
Consistency	Firm	Medium	Soft	
Position	Posterior	Mid	Anterior	

of contractions. Uterine overdistension will affect the conduct of labor and may be a factor in causing premature labor. This is frequently seen with multiple pregnancies, hydramnios, or fetal edema. It may be a problem at term for any of these reasons as well as because of an extremely large fetus. Uterine anatomy and volume are often factors in pathologic labor patterns; thus a bicornuate, didelphic, or unicornuate uterus may demonstrate abnormal uterine contraction patterns.

ARCHITECTURE OF THE BONY PELVIS

The seventh factor, the architecture of the bony pelvis, will be considered in detail in the next chapter.

ADDITIONAL READING

Bishop EH: Pelvic scoring for elective induction. *Obstet Gynecol* 1964; 24:260.

Cunningham FG, MacDonald PC, Gant NF: Attitude, lie, presentation and position of the fetus, in *Williams Obstetrics,* ed 18. E Norwalk, Conn, Appleton Lange, 1989.

Cunningham FG, MacDonald PC, Gant NF: Parturition: Biomolecular and physiologic processes, in *Williams Obstetrics,* ed 18. E Norwalk, Conn, Appleton Lange, 1989.

O'Brien WF, Cefalo RC: Labor and delivery, in Gabbe SG, Niebyl JR, Simpson JL (eds): *Obstetrics,* ed 2. New York, Churchill Livingstone, 1991.

Seeds JW: Malpresentations, in Gabbe SG, Niebyl JR, Simpson JL (eds): *Obstetrics,* ed 2. New York, Churchill Livingstone, 1991.

Weingold AB: The management of breech presentations, in Iffy L, Charles D (eds): *Operative Perinatology.* New York, Macmillan, 1984.

PELVIC ARCHITECTURE 3

All pelves may be separated, according to Caldwell and Moloy, into four classes:

1. Gynecoid
2. Android
3. Anthropoid
4. Platypelloid

The obstetrician uses this classification system to describe the configuration of the pelvis and its usable volume. The system is extremely practical since each pelvis shape has its own prognosis for labor.

While the Caldwell-Moloy classification designates these four "pure" pelvis types and while many pelves are indeed of the pure type, various mixtures of the basic configurations may also be found. Drawing a line through the greatest transverse diameter of the pelvic inlet divides the pelvis into anterior and posterior segments. With reference to descent of the fetus in labor, the pelvis may be further divided into planes: the planes of the pelvic inlet, the midpelvis, and the pelvic outlet. The posterior pelvic segment determines the basic type. The anterior segment demonstrates the variations. For example, a pelvis may be termed gynecoid-android in type, that is, a gynecoid pelvis with android tendencies. The importance of this classification is to provide an immediate three-dimensional picture of the pelvic planes and usable volume so that pathologic mechanisms of labor can be predicted and properly managed.

GYNECOID PELVIS

The gynecoid pelvis (Figure 3–1) is the most common type. Viewed through the inlet, it appears round or slightly ellipsoid. The transverse diameter of the inlet is only slightly longer than the anteroposterior dimension, and most of the area of the inlet is therefore usable space for the fetal head. The pubic arch is wide and allows the placement of two fingers side by side just beneath the symphysis. The sidewalls are parallel. Seen through the inlet, the pelvis resembles a cylinder without any narrowing from inlet to outlet.

Other characteristics of a gynecoid pelvis include a broad, well-rounded sacrosciatic notch and a sacrospinous ligament 2½ fingerbreadths in length. The ischial spines are barely palpable through the pelvic soft tissue and do not protrude into the birth canal. A mobile coccyx that bends out of the way as the head descends and a hollow, curved sacrum are present. The space between the ischial tuberosities (the intertuberous diameter) should accept the full breadth of a fist.

The gynecoid pelvis may be further described as large, average, or small, but it will have the identifying configuration outlined above. Since it is essentially round in shape,

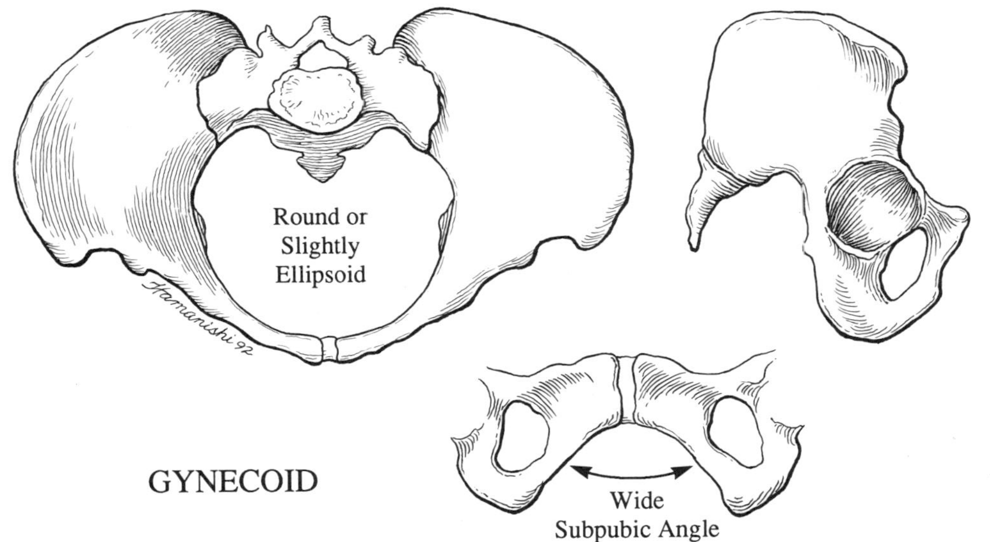

FIG 3–1.
Structural characteristics of a gynecoid pelvis.

the measurement of the anteroposterior diameter (conjugate diagonal) will give a rough picture of the inlet area. The conjugate diagonal is the distance from the lower margin of the pubic symphysis to the promontory of the sacrum. It is measured by placing the fingers of the examining hand against the lower border of the symphysis and pressing inward to reach the sacral promontory. The length is then measured on a ruler in centimeters. By subtracting 1.5 cm, the width of the pubic symphysis, we can arrive at the true inlet diameter. In practice, the measurement of the conjugate diagonal is somewhat uncomfortable for the patient. As experience is gained in performing pelvic examinations, this clinical estimate becomes a valuable tool for the physician in the diagnosis of potential cephalopelvic disproportion.

The following measurements represent a range often seen in gynecoid pelves. They are given primarily for the student's general information.

Pelvic inlet	
Transverse diameter	11.5–12.5cm
True conjugate (anteroposterior)	10.5–11.5cm
Midpelvis	
Interspinous diameter	10.0–11.0cm
Pelvic outlet	
Intertuberous diameter	9.5–10.5cm

ANDROID PELVIS

The android, or "male-like," pelvis (Fig 3–2) occurs less commonly than the gynecoid shape.

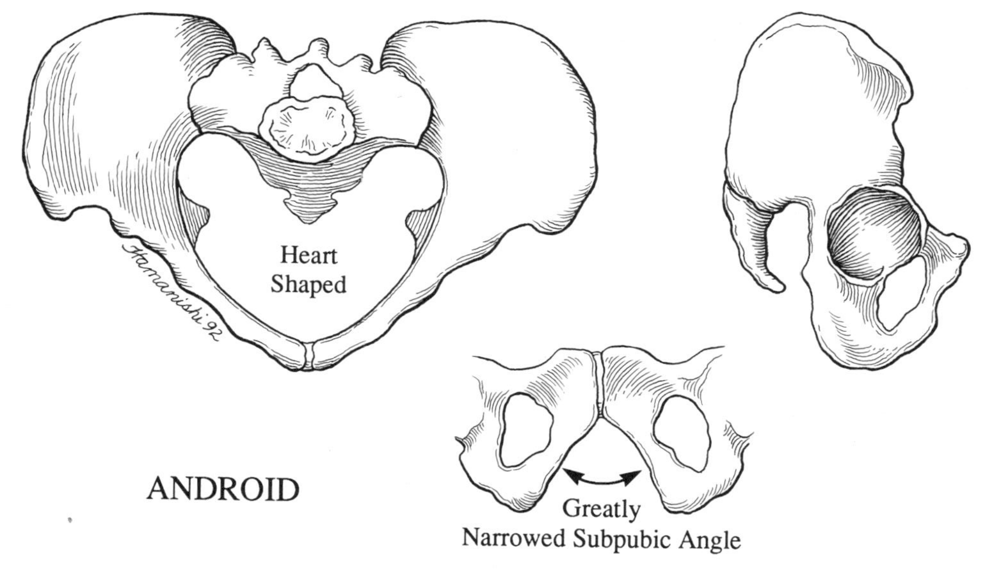

FIG 3–2.
Structural characteristics of an android pelvis.

An android pelvis is characterized by a posterior segment compromised in area by a forward-jutting sacral promontory and by a relatively long anterior segment. Viewed from a point above the pelvis, the plane of the inlet appears heart shaped. This configuration of the anterior and posterior segments limits usable pelvic volume. The bones of an android pelvis are generally heavy, so available space for descent is further limited.

At the level of the midpelvis in the pure android type, usable volume further decreases. The pelvic sidewalls converge rather than remaining parallel as in the gynecoid configuration. The ishial spines are very prominent, protrude into the birth canal, and can be easily identified on pelvic examination. The sacrosciatic notch is narrowed and highly arched, and the sacrospinous ligaments are less than 2½ fingerbreadths in length.

Examination of the outlet plane reveals a greatly narrowed pubic arch, one of the important identifying features of the android classification. The student will find the he can barely place one finger beneath the pubis. The sacrum is frequently angulated rather than curved or hollow, which further limits space. The intertuberous diameter is narrowed and accommodates a clenched fist poorly, if at all, on examination.

ANTHROPOID PELVIS

The anthropoid pelvis (Fig 3–3) has a striking oval shape at the plane of the pelvic inlet, with the largest diameter of

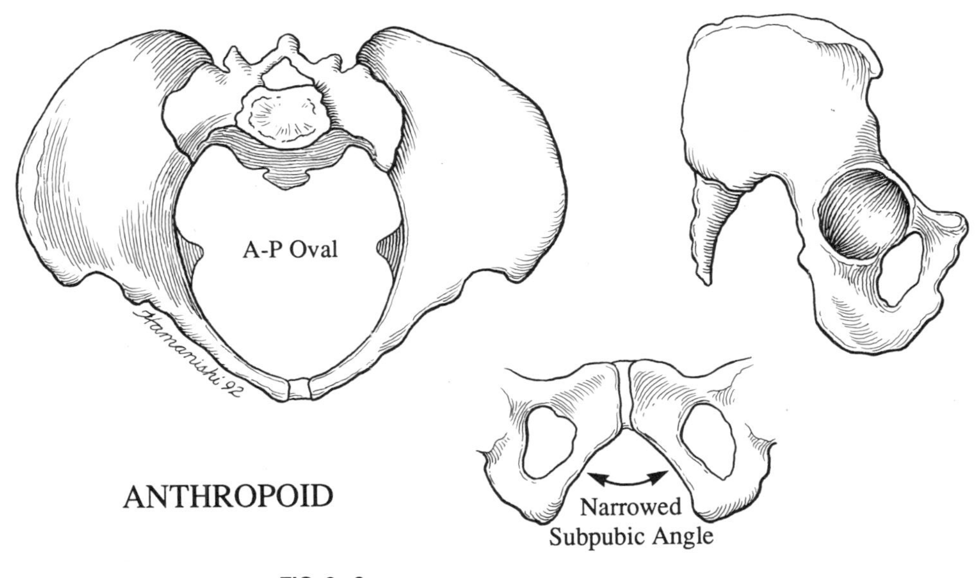

FIG 3–3.
Structural characteristics of an anthropoid pelvis.

the oval in the anteroposterior dimension. The posterior segment is therefore long and narrow. Engagement must occur with the long axis of the fetal skull perpendicular to the transverse diameter of the inlet.

At the plane of the midpelvis the majority of anthropoid pelves show parallel sidewalls, although some demonstrate convergence. The prominence of the spines may be real or seemingly so because the midpelvis is narrow. The sacrosciatic notch is very wide, more so than in a gynecoid pelvis. The sacrum is frequently elongated and may contain as many as six vertebrae.

The pubic arch is narrow and less than two fingerbreadths wide, thus causing outlet contraction. Anthropoid pelves, however, are often large and frequently do not interfere with vaginal delivery. More likely they will be associated with an abnormal labor pattern because in the majority of instances the fetus will engage in the posterior presentation. Of those few (perhaps 10%) instances where the fetus engages in the vertex anterior presentation, labor may be extremely rapid.

PLATYPELLOID PELVIS

A platypelloid pelvis (Fig 3–4) is flat with delicate bones. It is the least common pure pelvic type and is found in fewer than 3% of patients.

Most striking in the platypelloid pelvis is the inlet configuration, which demonstrates extreme flattening in the an-

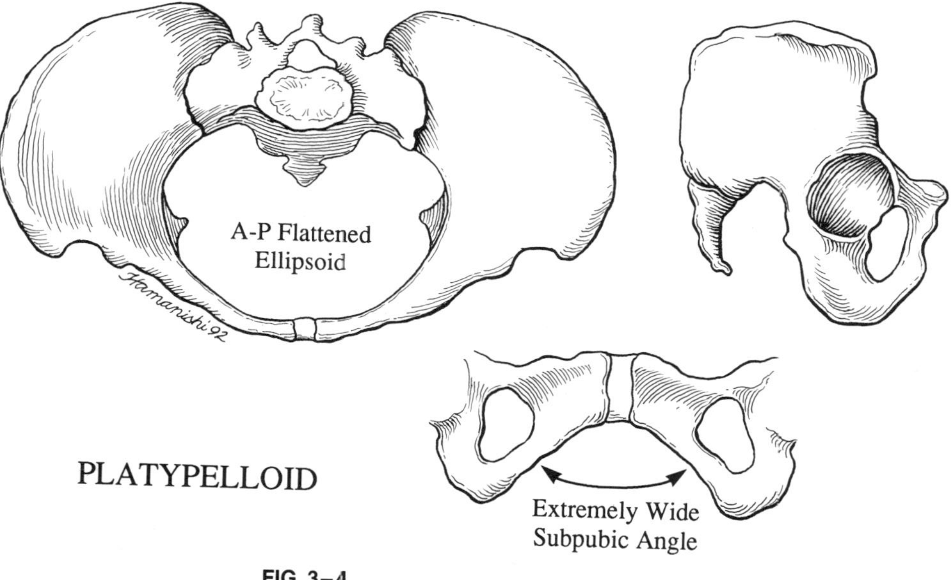

FIG 3–4.
Structural characteristics of a platypelloid pelvis.

teroposterior diameter in contrast to a wide transverse measurement. The findings on examination are a short conjugate diameter, a wide posterior segment, and a flattened, ellipsoid appearance when viewed from above.

The sidewalls are generally straight. Midpelvic contraction is not a problem in a pure platypelloid pelvis. Since the pubic arch is extremely wide and the sacrum short and deviated posteriorly, outlet dystocia is not common.

Because of its unusual inlet diameters, an average platypelloid pelvis may have a profound effect on the conduct of normal labor. The mechanism of engagement is usually in the transverse rather than the anteroposterior attitude, and the size of the fetus is a critical factor in vaginal delivery. Usable pelvic volume, as in android and, more particularly, anthropoid pelves, is most compromised at the inlet.

ADDITIONAL READING

Cunningham FG, MacDonald PC, Gant NF: Dystocia due to pelvic contraction, in *Williams Obstetrics,* ed 18. E Norwalk, Conn, Appleton-Lange, 1989.

Cunningham FG, MacDonald PC, Gant NF: The normal pelvis, in *Williams Obstetrics,* ed 18. E Norwalk, Conn, Appleton-Lange, 1989.

O'Brien WF, Cefalo RC: Labor and delivery, in Gabbe SG, Niebyl JR, Simpson JL (eds): *Obstetrics,* ed 2. New York, Churchill Livingstone, 1991.

THE LABOR CURVE 4

The progress of labor may be plotted on a graph. Most normal labors follow a curve described by Friedman, which will be discussed here in some detail. Knowledge of the curve and how labor should proceed along it make it possible to detect abnormalities of labor in a relatively early stage.

In general, the patient's general medical condition, her pelvic architecture, the size, position, and presentation of the fetus, the strength of uterine contractions, and the softness and effacement of the cervix will influence the progress of the labor as depicted by the labor curve. Knowing several of these factors in advance may make it possible for the physician to predict the type of labor the patient may have and therefore anticipate problems that may occur and interventions that may be necessary.

Figure 4–1 depicts the Friedman curve, which relates the dilatation of the cervix to time 0, or that time at which regular meaningful contractions occur. The curve is plotted with cervical dilatation (in centimeters) on the vertical axis and increments of time on the horizontal axis. The time in

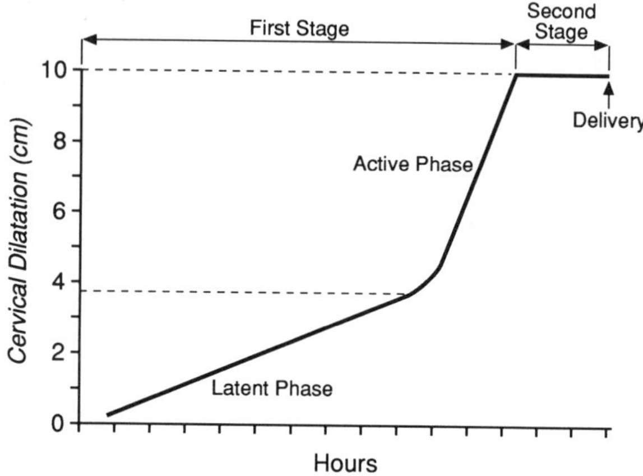

FIG 4–1.
The course of normal labor may be illustrated on a graph where cervical dilatation is plotted against time. The major components of the resulting curve are the first stage, which includes the latent and accelerated phases of labor, and the second stage, which extends from the time that the cervix becomes fully dilated to the moment the baby is delivered. This curve is useful because of its diagnostic, therapeutic, and prognostic implications, which render it a practical clinical device. The components of the curve are further useful for descriptive purposes and may assist in determining the motive and timing of obstetric interference. The physician should picture the curve each time he/she follows a patient in labor to thereby gain insight into the pathologic processes that may arise.

labor will (1) vary in inverse relation to parity, (2) vary depending on compromise of the factors of normal labor, and (3) give an indication as to the method and moment of interference in abnormal labor patterns that may benefit the patient.

Note that the curve may be divided into several segments: the first stage of labor, which comprises the latent phase and the accelerated, or active, phase, and the second stage, which occurs from the time of full dilatation until delivery of the baby. The third stage of labor is that time between the delivery of the fetus and the delivery of the placenta.

LATENT PHASE

The latent phase of labor, represented by the first segment of the curve, is marked by the onset of uterine contractions. It involves dilatation of the cervix from 0 to about 3 cm. Since some patients enter labor more dilated than 0, cervical dilatation is generally measured from that point of entry until 3 cm. During this time effacement of the cervix is completed. This period may be thought of as a time when the forces concerned with normal labor are being coordinated. In a vertex presentation the fetal head descends into the pelvis. When relative or absolute disproportion is present, some early molding with caput formation may occur.

The latent phase is generally measured in hours, its length of duration depending on several circumstances. If complete or nearly complete and effacement has occurred when contractions begin, the latent phase will be shortened. If uterine contractions begin with the cervix poorly effaced and the presenting part at a high station, a relatively long latent phase may be expected. By itself this is not necessarily pathologic.

Through improper management the latent phase of labor may be prolonged. Heavy sedation during this period of time, amniotomy, or at times the application of conduction anesthesia in the form of a caudal or an epidural may cause a prolongation of this phase. Contractions during the latent phase are mild in quality, but depending on the patient's pain threshold, may be experienced as very painful. Fear and anxiety may also act to extend the latent phase. Often mild sedation to relieve the patient's anxiety may be helpful in shortening the latent phase, and when necessary, intravenous oxytocin can be used.

ACCELERATED, OR ACTIVE, PHASE

The second portion of the first stage of labor is noted on the labor curve as a steep change in slope and is referred to as the accelerated phase. When cervical dilatation proceeds in this manner, the patient is said to be in active labor. Time in active labor may be measured in hours in a primigravida or in a patient with an abnormal presentation or in minutes with some grand multiparas.

Characteristics of the accelerated phase include (1) regular contractions of good quality and (2) progress in labor as determined by dilatation and descent. In vertex presentations the presenting part descends into the pelvis, becomes applied to the cervix, and acts as an efficient dilating wedge. Amniotomy during this phase may be desirable and is usually technically simple. It will generally shorten the time in labor, but many authorities prefer to leave the membranes intact until nearly full dilatation. Medication in the form of analgesia and mild sedation may be given during this phase and generally will have no effect on lengthening of the time course of the active phase. Gentle examinations and encouragement on the part of the physician are, of course, welcome.

The period of time required to complete the accelerated phase, that is, from 3 cm to full dilatation, averages 5 hours for a primigravida and 2.2 hours for a multipara. In comparison, the latent phase averages 8.6 and 5.3 hours, respectively.

SECOND STAGE OF LABOR

After full dilatation the patient is in the second stage of labor. During this phase the vertex will generally rotate to an occipitoanterior position and complete its descent to the perineum. When it bulges the perineum, it is known to be crowning, and from then on delivery can be effected either spontaneously or with the help of vacuum extraction or forceps delivery. Therefore, the length of time of the second stage of labor depends on the patient's ability to push the presenting part to a point where it is deliverable and whether or not delivery is assisted by either forceps or vacuum extraction; it is somewhat longer if assisting methods are not utilized.

The Mechanism of Labor

To further understand the labor curve, let us briefly consider the mechanisms of labor in the vertex presentation along with some illustrative examples of variance from the course of normal labor.

The following mechanism of labor is for the vertex presentation and occurs in all pelvic types in the absence of absolute cephalopelvic disproportion. When labor begins, descent of the vertex proceeds until the phenomenon of engagement occurs. Engagement of the vertex is present when the widest diameter (biparietal diameter) of the vertex has passed the plane of the pelvic inlet. The determination of engagement is of importance in labor. However, since we cannot palpate the pelvic brim and its relation to the biparietal diameter, engagement is determined indirectly. The distance from the pelvic inlet to the ischial spines is about 5 cm. Therefore, we record engagement when the vertex has descended to the level of the ischial spines and assume that the major volume of the presenting part has passed the plane of the inlet. When the presenting part is at the level of the ischial spines, its station is said to be zero. Stations above the spines are referred to as minus stations and are given in centimeters (i.e., −1, −2, −3). Those below the spines are referred to as plus stations (i.e., +1, +2, +3) (Fig 4–2). In gynecoid pelves engagement generally occurs in an occipitotransverse position with subsequent rotation to occipitoanterior. In narrow pelves engagement usually occurs in the occipitoposterior position but may occasionally occur in the occipitoanterior position. Engagement in platypelloid pelves must occur in occipitotransverse positions because of the shortened conjugate diagonal.

Descent, flexion, and internal rotation to the occipitoanterior position occurs following engagement. The vertex approaches the pelvic floor, and distension and flattening of

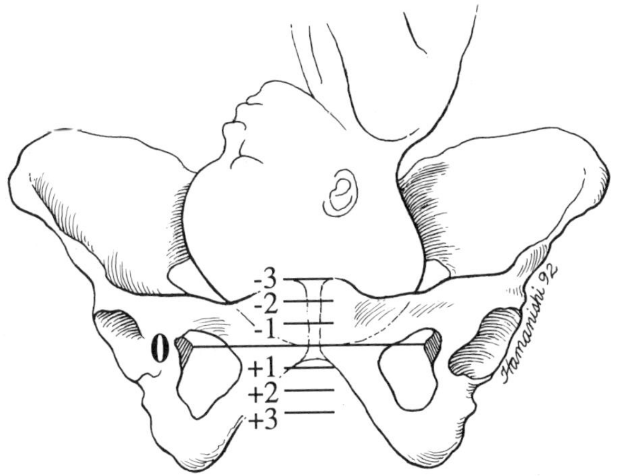

FIG 4–2.
Stations of the vertex with respect to the ischial spines.

the perineal muscles precede crowning of the infant's head. The occiput, forehead, nose, mouth, and chin are delivered by extension of the vertex over the posterior of the perineum (Fig 4–3). This is followed by spontaneous external rotation to the position that was present just prior to expulsion.

Delivery of the shoulders, body, and hindquarters follows, and the second stage of labor is ended (Figs 4–4 and 4–5). The cord is clamped and cut, and cord blood samples are obtained. The entire process of labor is terminated with the third stage, which involves delivery of the pla-

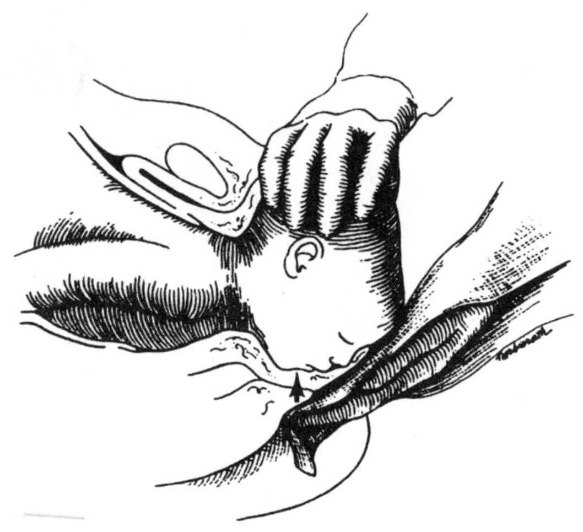

FIG 4–3.
Delivery of the head. (From Iffy L, Charles D: *Operative Perinatology*. New York, Macmillan, 1984. Used by permission.)

centa and inspection of the uterus, cervix, and vagina for any injuries that may have occurred.

The following are four examples of fetal-maternal relationships that may influence the pattern of the labor curve.

OCCIPITOPOSTERIOR POSITION IN A GYNECOID PELVIS

Prolongation of the accelerated (active) phase of labor will usually occur when the vertex descends in the occipitopos-

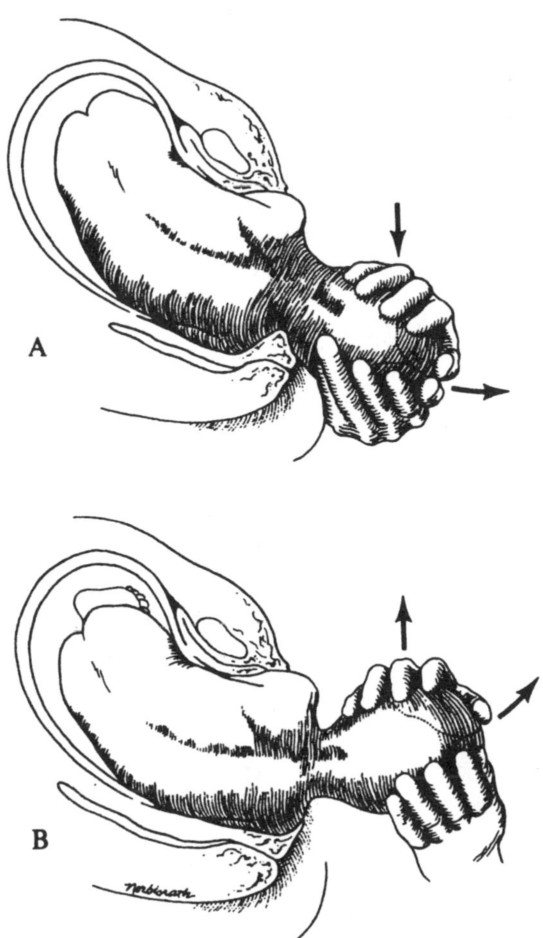

FIG 4–4.
Delivery of the shoulders. (From Iffy L, Charles D: *Operative Perinatology*. New York, Macmillan, 1984. Used by permission.)

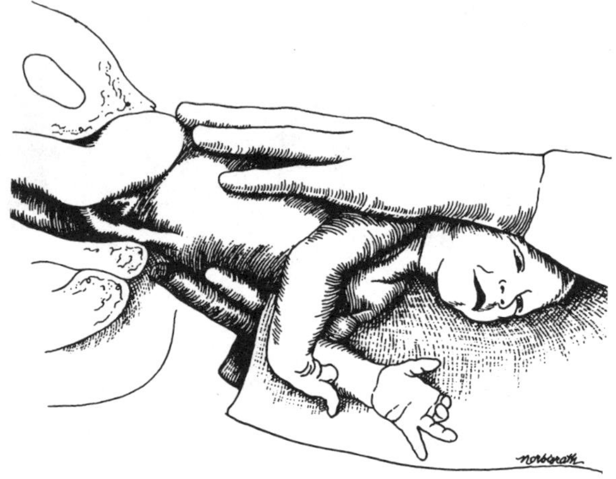

FIG 4–5.
Delivery of the body. (From Iffy L, Charles D: *Operative Perinatology*. New York, Macmillan, 1984. Used by permission.)

terior position. The vertex remains in a deflexed attitude until descent to the levator sling has been accomplished. Rotation of the occiput to the anterior position will then occur, and delivery by extension follows. Until the mechanism of internal rotation takes place, slowing of the labor progress at 7 to 9 cm may be encountered (Fig 4–6). This is referred to as "desultory labor in the posterior position," or "positional dystocia," and in selected cases can be corrected by oxytocin stimulation.

LABOR MECHANISMS IN A NARROW PELVIS

The vertex-posterior position is more common in android and anthropoid pelves. Owing to midpelvic contraction, prominent spines, and varying degrees of sidewall convergence typical of these pelvic types, descent and anterior rotation may be hampered or may not occur. A prolonged accelerated phase of labor usually results. This is reflected by a decrease in the slope of the labor curve.

The proper management of relative cephalopelvic disproportion depends upon the physician's ability to determine

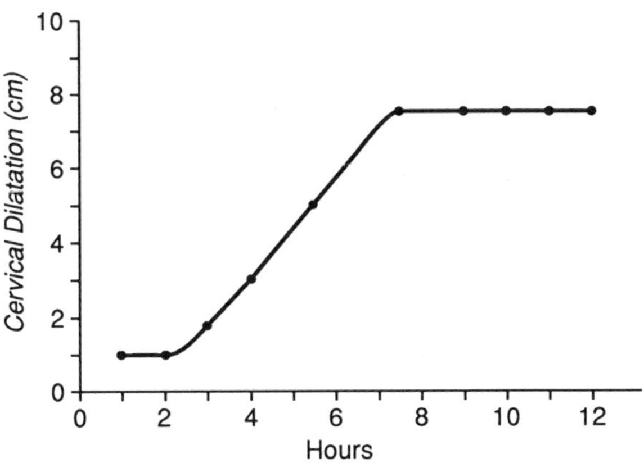

FIG 4–6.
Typical labor curve in an occipitoposterior presentation demonstrating slowing of the accelerated phase of labor at 7 cm.

the proximal cause of the positional dystocia. After careful evaluation of the patient, a diagnosis based on estimated fetal weight, position of the vertex, clinical pelvimetry performed during the vaginal examination, and quality and interval of uterine contractions should be recorded. Therapy in the form of general support, hydration, sedation, and oxytocin augmentation may allow progress to occur. When progress in dilatation and descent becomes arrested despite careful interference, abdominal delivery is indicated. Finally, it must be emphasized that throughout the course of prolonged labor careful attention should be given to the condition of the mother and the fetus in order to ensure a safe conduct of labor to delivery.

RAPID LABOR IN THE ACCELERATED PHASE

An anthropoid pelvis, although narrow at the inlet plane, has much usable volume in the anteroposterior direction. When engagement of the vertex occurs in the occipitoanterior position (approximately 10% of the cases), little bony obstruction is present, and rapid descent may occur. If contractions are of good quality, the accelerated phase of labor will be shortened, and rapid expulsion may follow. The consequences of precipitous delivery may include cervical lacerations with bleeding, deep vaginal or perineal tears, infant skull injury, and infant depression.

The labor curve illustrates this course (Fig 4–7). Obstetric intervention is directed toward control of progress of labor and management of crowning and expulsion. Adequate sedation will allow better evaluation of rapid labor and will

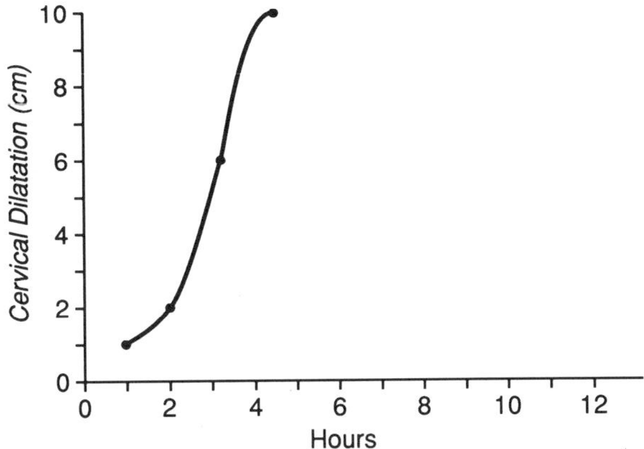

FIG 4–7.
Example of a rapid labor in a primigravida with an anthropoid pelvis and vertex engaged in the occipitoanterior position.

relieve anxiety that is frequently excessive. A most efficient method of control of rapid labor is the use of conduction anesthesia such as a caudal or an epidural. This will relieve pain, eliminate the expulsion reflex, and negate the force of abdominal muscle contractions. Under severe circumstances tocolytic agents may be used.

TRANSVERSE ARREST

Engagement and descent must occur in the occipitotransverse position in a platypelloid pelvis owing to the configuration of the inlet plane. Rotation to the anterior plane and flexion occur as the vertex reaches the levator sling.

Slowing of the accelerated phase of labor will be observed if rotation and flexion cannot occur because of pelvic contraction. With the occiput in a transverse position, arrest in labor results and necessitates stimulation with oxytocics. If failure of progression then occurs, abdominal delivery may be necessary, but in some situations the baby will descend in the transverse position and be delivered in that fashion. While forceps are available for application in the transverse presentation, i.e., Barton and Kjeland forceps, such maneuvers are generally not necessary.

ADDITIONAL READING

Cunningham FG, MacDonald PC, Gant NF: Conduct of normal labor and delivery, in *Williams Obstetrics,* ed 18. E Norwalk, Conn, Appleton Lange, 1989.

Cunningham FG, MacDonald PC, Gant NF: Mechanisms of normal labor in occipital presentation, in *Williams Obstetrics,* ed 18. E Norwalk, Conn, Appleton Lange, 1989.

Friedman EA: *Labor: Clinical Evaluation and Management,* ed 2. New York, Appleton, 1978.

O'Brien WF, Cefalo RC: Labor and delivery, in Gabbe SG, Niebyl JL, Simpson JL (eds): *Obstetrics,* ed 2. New York, Churchill Livingstone, 1991.

Stenchever MA: Normal vaginal delivery, in Iffy L, Charles D (eds): *Operative Perinatology*. New York, Macmillan, 1984.

INTRAPARTUM MONITORING 5

Assessment of the fetal heart rate allows intrapartum evaluation of fetal well-being. Intermittent auscultation of fetal heart tones is adequate in an uncomplicated low-risk pregnancy; high-risk pregnancies require continuous electronic fetal heart rate monitoring. This can be accomplished with a pulsed Doppler ultrasound transducer placed on the maternal abdomen over the uterus or with an electrode placed directly in fetal skin following rupture of the membranes (Fig 5–1). Direct monitoring, although more invasive, provides more detailed and accurate information (Fig 5–2). In patients with human immunodeficiency virus or herpes simplex virus, electrodes are avoided because they provide a direct port of entry for the virus to the fetus.

MONITORING METHODS

Intermittent auscultation has been used successfully to detect fetal distress in low-risk pregnancies (Table 5–1). A fetal stethoscope or Doppler ultrasound transducer is used to ascertain the fetal heart rate every 15 minutes during the first stage of labor and every 5 minutes in the second stage. For a patient to qualify for intermittent rather than continuous monitoring, some obstetric units require an ini-

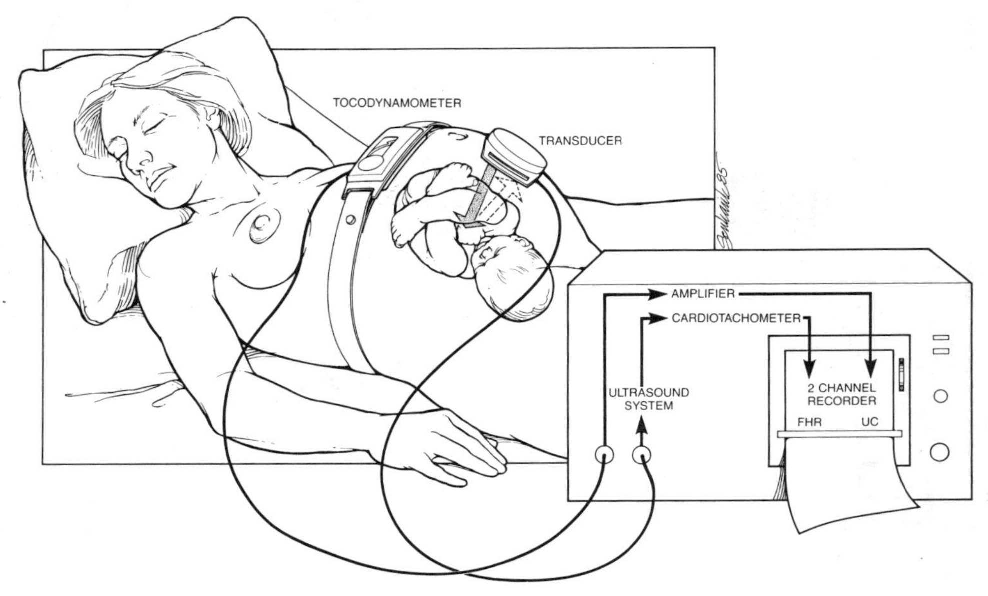
TOCODYNAMOMETER
TRANSDUCER
AMPLIFIER
CARDIOTACHOMETER
ULTRASOUND
SYSTEM
2 CHANNEL
RECORDER
FHR
UC

TABLE 5–1.
Intermittent Monitoring

Stage	Monitoring
On admission to the labor ward	Perform a nonstress test
First stage of labor	Check fetal heart tones every 15 min
Second stage of labor	Check fetal heart tones with each contraction

tial normal continuous heart rate tracing for 20 minutes, while other units require only examination of amniotic fluid for the absence of meconium. Intermittent monitoring is usually carried out after a contraction for 1 minute at a time, although some clinicians prefer to monitor during a contraction. If the heart rate is <100 or >160 beats per minute (bpm) during or after three contractions, further evaluation with continuous monitoring or fetal scalp pH determinations (see below) is indicated.

With continuous fetal monitoring, it is necessary to simultaneously record uterine activity in relation to the fetal heart rate. A strain gauge may be placed externally over the uterus to measure the change in myometrial tone with

FIG 5–1.
External fetal monitors. (From Gabbe SG, Niebyl JR, Simpson JL: *Obstetrics*. New York, Churchill Livingstone, 1986. Used by permission.)

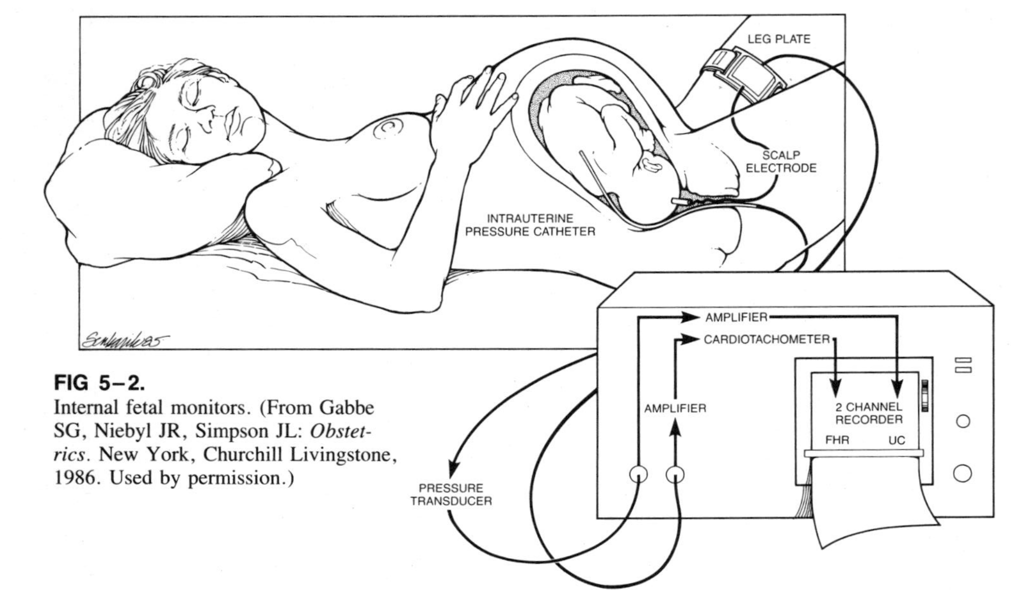

FIG 5–2.
Internal fetal monitors. (From Gabbe SG, Niebyl JR, Simpson JL: *Obstetrics*. New York, Churchill Livingstone, 1986. Used by permission.)

contractions. Alternatively, the gauge may be attached to the end of a water-filled catheter inserted directly into the uterus. Only the intrauterine pressure catheter allows a determination of the strength of contractions, but the timing of contractions can be assessed with either method.

PHYSIOLOGY OF THE FETAL HEART RATE

The physiology of the fetal heart rate is quite different from that of the adult. In the fetus, the Starling mechanism is poorly developed; the fetus has little ability to increase stroke volume with increased preload. Fetal cardiac output thus depends primarily on the heart rate. A variety of factors influence the fetal heart rate. The fetal heart is under tonic sympathetic (Fig 5–3) and parasympathetic control (Fig 5–4). The parasympathetic (vagal) influence decreases the intrinsic heart rate, and tonic sympathetic discharge increases the fetal heart rate. The vagal nerve also transmits impulses responsible for fetal heart rate variability. Heart rate variability is a complex but important aspect of fetal evaluation since normal variability reflects normal cerebral oxygenation. The sympathetic nervous system is responsible for redistribution of fetal blood flow to the brain and vital organs in times of stress.

Fetal chemoreceptors (Fig 5–5) and baroreceptors (Fig 5–6) also interact to control the heart rate. Central chemoreceptors cause an increased heart rate and hypertension in response to hypoxia or hypercapnia, while pe-

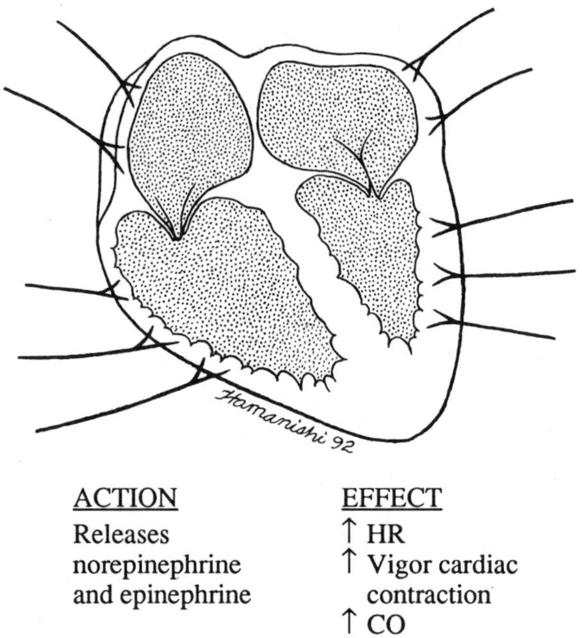

FIG 5–3.
Sympathetic innervation. (*HR* = heart rate; *CO* = cardiac output).

ripheral chemoreceptors cause bradycardia. Stimulation of baroreceptors by hypertension also causes bradycardia. The combination of these influences generally results in fetal bradycardia following hypoxia and asphyxia. However, tachycardia may also indicate fetal distress.

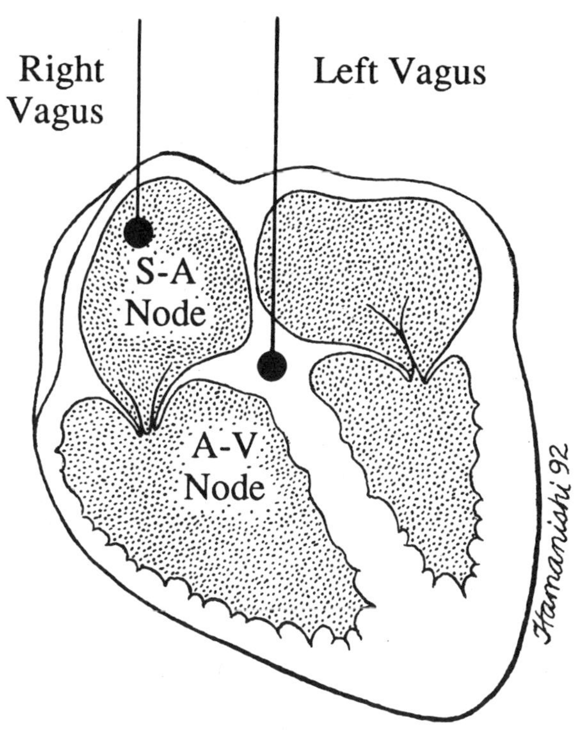

ACTION	EFFECT
Releases acetylcholine	↓ HR Transmits variability

FIG 5–4.
Parasympathetic innvervation. (*HR* = heart rate.)

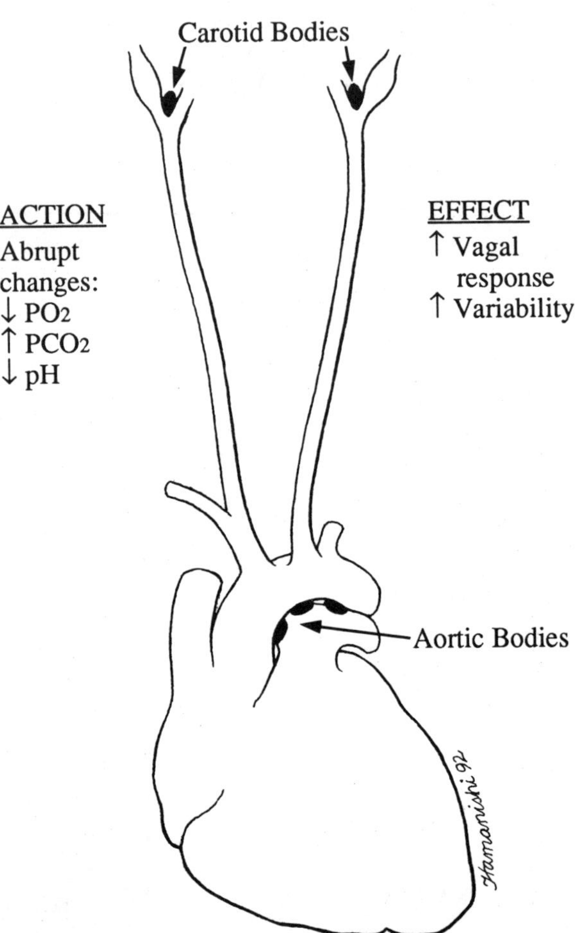

FIG 5–5.
Peripheral chemoreceptors.

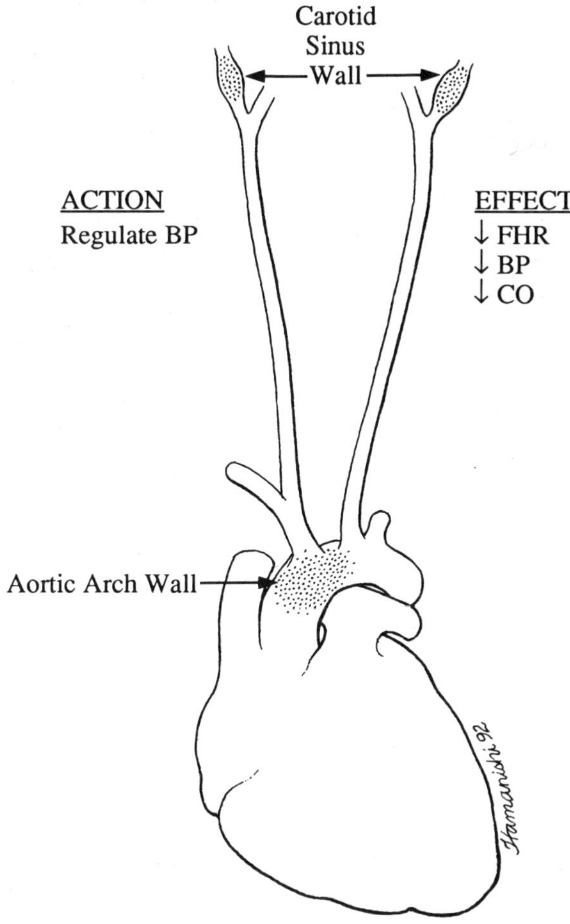

FIG 5–6.
Baroreceptors. (*BP* = blood pressure; *FHR* = fetal heart rate; *CO* = cardiac output.)

FEATURES OF FETAL HEART RATE TRACINGS

Every fetal heart rate tracing should be assessed methodically (Tables 5–2 and 5–3). The important features are the baseline fetal heart rate, variability, and periodic change. The baseline rate normally lies between 120 and 160 bpm and decreases with increasing gestational age be-

TABLE 5–2.

Fetal Heart Rate Abnormalities and Their Etiologies

Bradycardia
Fetal hypoxia
Placental hypoperfusion
Drug effect (β-blocker)
Heart block
Tachycardia
Maternal fever
Chorioamniolitis
Drug effect
Supraventricular tachycardia
Asphyxia
Recovery phase after bradycardia
Decreased variability
Extreme prematurity
Hypoxia
Narcotics
β-Blockers
Fetal sleep state
Decelerations
Early deceleration: Head compression
Variable deceleration: Cord compression
Late deceleration: Hypoxia, hypoperfusion, myocardial depression

TABLE 5–3.
Features of Fetal Heart Rate Tracing

- Baseline
- Variability
  - Short-term
  - Long-term
- Periodic changes
  - Accelerations
  - Decelerations
    - Early
    - Variable
      - Mild
      - Moderate
      - Severe
    - Late

cause of increasing vagal tone. Bradycardia (Fig 5–7) may be the fetal response to hypoxia or uteroplacental hypoperfusion (asphyxia) or may be due to a drug effect (e.g., β-adrenergic antagonists). A rare cause of fetal bradycardia is heart block, most often seen in conjunction with structural cardiac disease or in fetuses of mothers with systemic lupus erythematosus. Fetal tachycardia is commonly due to increased maternal temperature, chorioamnionitis, drug effect, or tachyarrhythmias such as supraventricular tachycardia. Tachycardia may also be seen in asphyxia or in the recovery phase after bradycardia.

The small transient increases and decreases in the baseline fetal heart rate are called variability (Fig 5–8). Variability is categorized as short-term or long-term. Short-term vari-

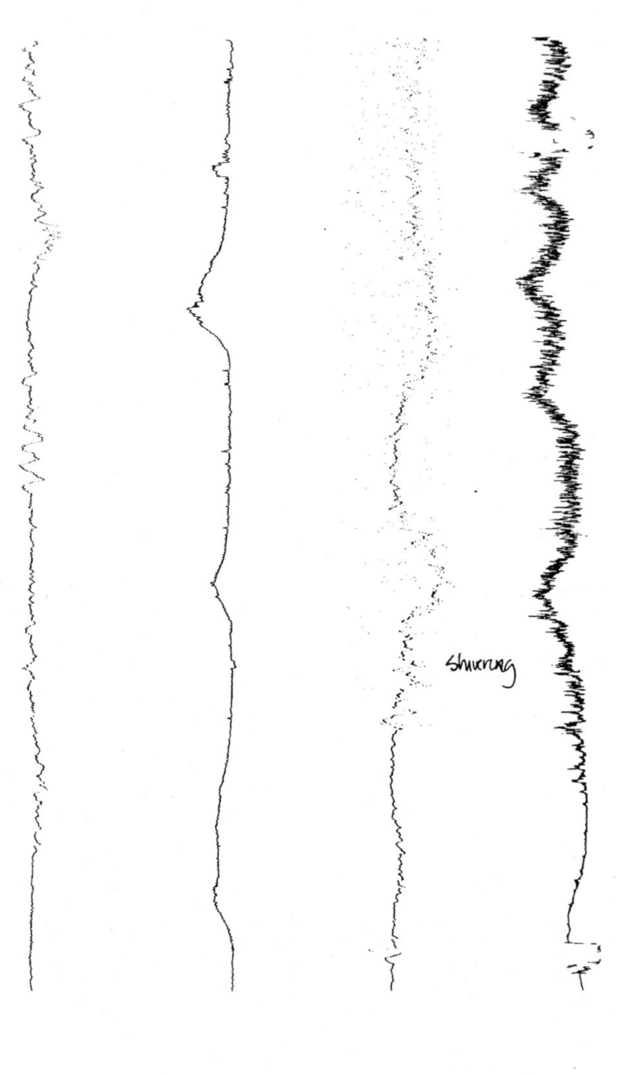
shivering

ability occurs "beat to beat," while long-term variability is seen as oscillations of about 6 bpm occurring three to five times per minute. Variability increases with fetal maturation and may be decreased in very young fetuses (<30 weeks). Variability is decreased with hypoxia (Fig 5–9). Some drugs, especially β-adrenergic blockers, also decrease variability. Exaggerated long-term variability, often referred to as a "saltatory" pattern, is benign unless accompanied or followed by other abnormal patterns such as bradycardia. When short-term variability is absent and the heart rate has a sinusoidal variation, fetal anemia or a narcotic effect should be suspected.

Periodic changes in the fetal heart rate include accelerations and decelerations. Accelerations are a sign of fetal well-being and occur in response to fetal stimulation such as fetal movement, uterine contraction, scalp stimulation, or acoustic stimulation. A fetus is said to be "reactive" if accelerations of at least 15 bpm above baseline lasting at least 15 seconds are present (Fig 5–10). As with variability, fetal maturity influences reactivity; very early fetuses may not demonstrate accelerations. The absence of accelerations (a "nonreactive" tracing) does not necessarily imply fetal distress but must be evaluated in the context of other heart rate and clinical features.

FIG 5–7.
Bradycardia. (From Schifrin BS: *Exercises in fetal monitoring,* vol 1. Los Angeles, BPM, 1990. Used by permission.)

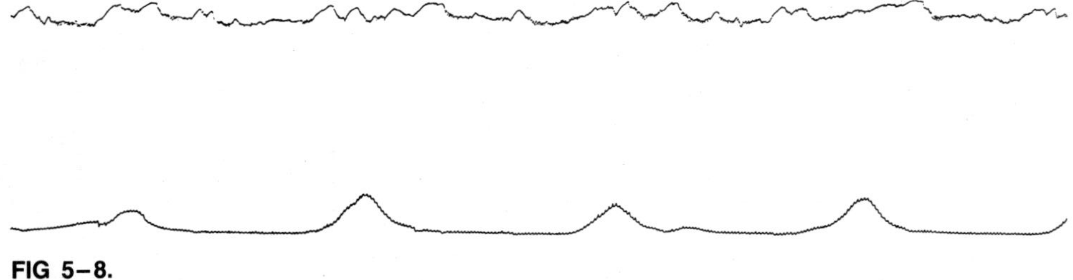

FIG 5–8.
Normal variability. (From Schifrin BS: *Exercises in Fetal Monitoring*, vol 1. Los Angeles, BPM, 1990. Used by permission.)

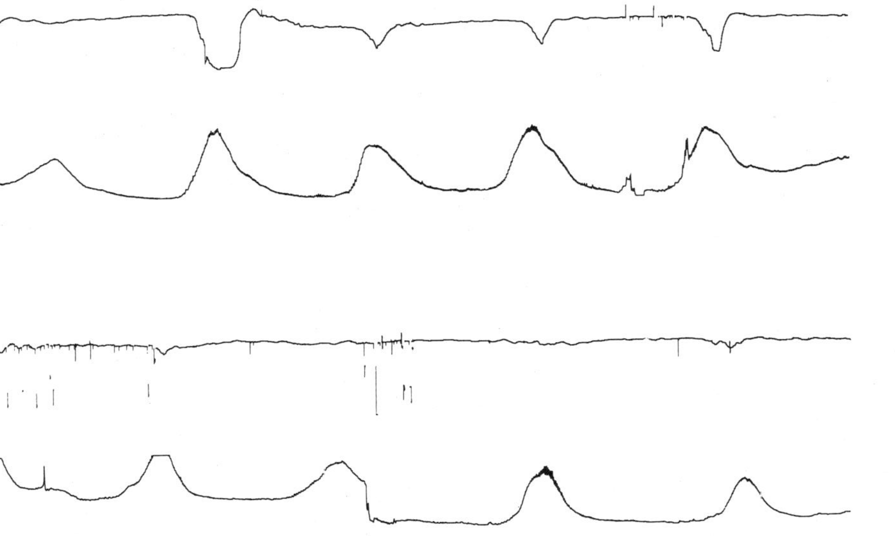

FIG 5–9.
Decreased variability. (From Schifrin BS: *Exercises in Fetal Monitoring*, vol 1. Los Angeles, BPM, 1990. Used by permission.)

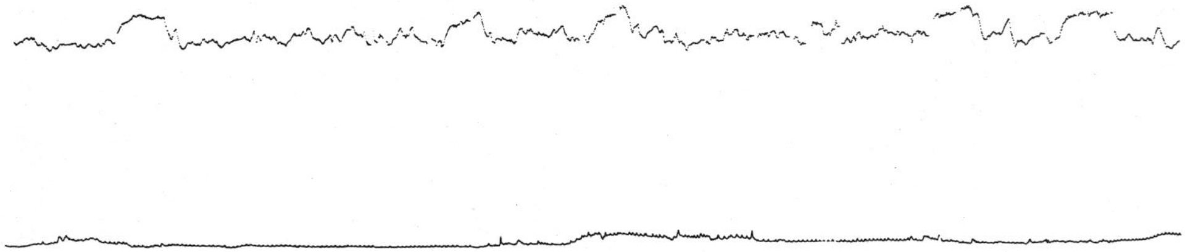

FIG 5–10.
Reactivity. (From Schifrin BS: *Exercises in Fetal Monitoring,* vol 1. Los Angeles, BPM, 1990. Used by permission.)

Decelerations of the fetal heart rate are common during labor. They may be "early," "late," or "variable." Early decelerations occur with fetal head compression and are smooth, gentle, and shallow (less than 20 bpm). They begin and end at the same time as a contraction and are considered benign. Late decelerations (Fig 5–11) are similar in shape to early decelerations but begin after the start of a contraction and end after the contraction ends. This pattern is ominous and usually reflects fetal hypoxia or hypoperfusion. When variability and accelerations are absent, late decelerations may even indicate direct myocardial depression (Fig 5–12). The third deceleration pattern, variable deceleration, is due to umbilical cord compression (Fig 5–13). This pattern is recognized by a sudden drop in fetal heart rate with the onset of a contraction and an abrupt return to normal as the uterus relaxes. In an otherwise healthy fetus, mild variable decelerations are well tolerated. However, severe variable decelerations meeting "60-60-60" criteria (below 60 bpm, decreasing more than 60 bpm, or lasting longer than 60 seconds) can indicate impending or actual fetal acidosis.

In summary, fetal compromise should be suspected when there is a combination of any of the following patterns present on the fetal heart rate tracing: increased or decreased baseline rate, absent or markedly decreased variability, lack of reactivity, or late or severe variable decelerations. In practice, other conditions such as meconium staining of amniotic fluid, maternal illness, fetal growth, amniotic fluid volume, and gestational age must also be considered. Prenatal history is often essential in clinical decision making.

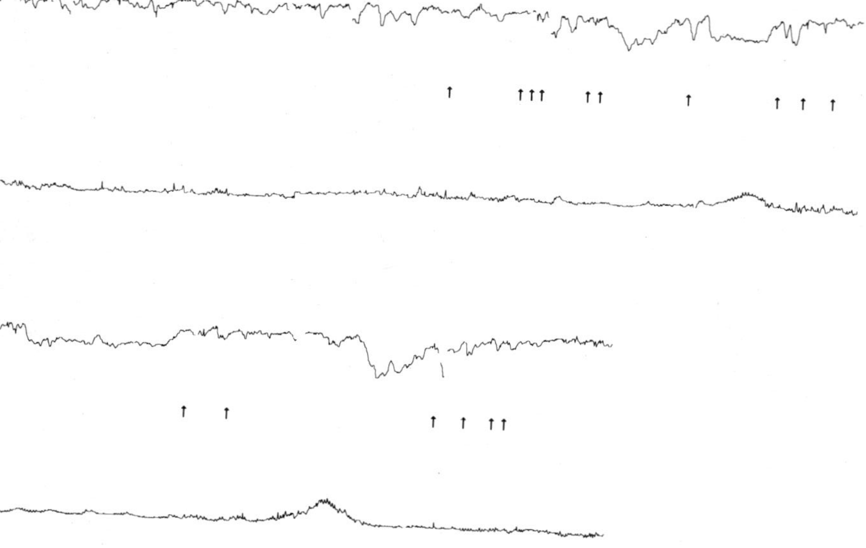

FIG 5–11.
Late deceleration. (From Schifrin BS: *Exercises in Fetal Monitoring*, vol 3. Los Angeles, BPM, 1990. Used by permission.)

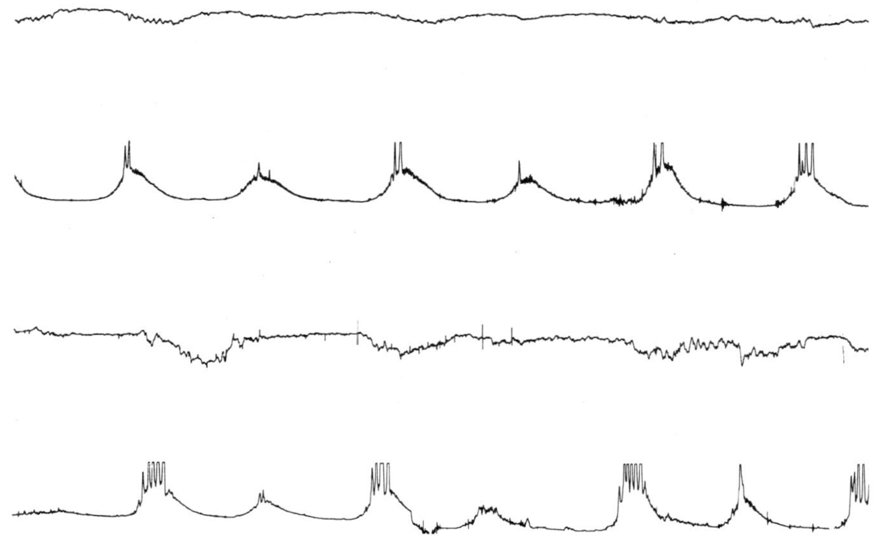

FIG 5–12.
Late deceleration with decreased variability. (From Schifrin BS: *Exercises in Fetal Monitoring*, vol 1. Los Angeles, BPM, 1990. Used by permission.)

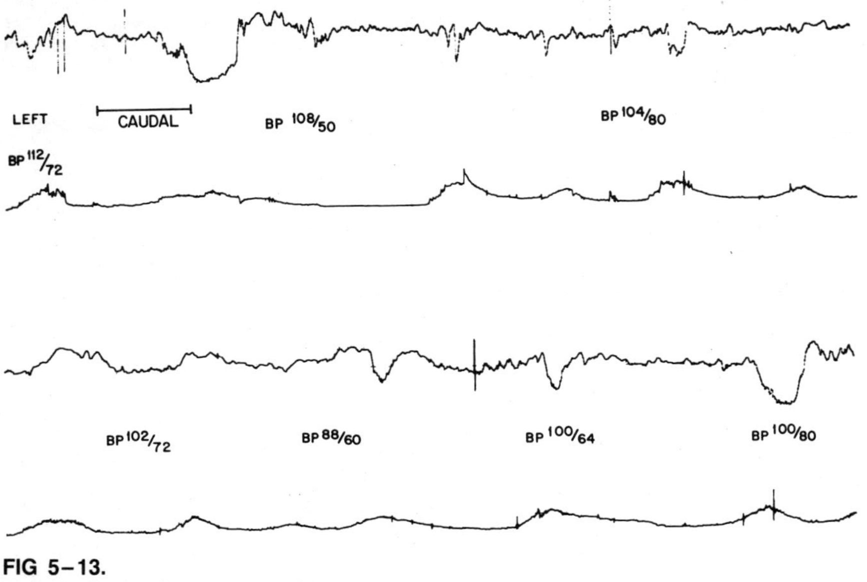

FIG 5–13.
Variable decelerations. (From Schifrin BS: *Exercises in Fetal Monitoring*, vol 1. Los Angeles, BPM, 1990. Used by permission.)

Ideally, the underlying cause of distress should be determined and corrected, but in practice this is not always possible. Causes of fetal compromise include uterine hypoperfusion due to maternal hypotension, intrinsic abnormal placental function, placental separation, cord compression, and an abnormal fetus. Some of these causes can be treated only with immediate delivery; others respond to conservative measures.

FETAL COMPROMISE AND DISTRESS

A number of measures should be routinely employed in the diagnosis and management of an abnormal fetal heart rate (Table 5–4). First, the maternal vital signs are determined; hypotension due to medication or a regional anesthetic is a frequent cause of fetal bradycardia due to uterine hypoperfusion. The maternal position should be changed, especially if supine hypotension from vena caval compression by the uterus is suspected. If oxytocin is being used, it should be discontinued, and if uterine hyperstimulation is present, tocolytic therapy should be considered. Decreasing contractions can maximize uteroplacental

TABLE 5–4.
Scalp pH Measurements

pH	Management
>7.25	Follow the fetal heart rate pattern closely
7.20–7.25	Repeat scalp pH immediately
<7.20	Perform cesarean section if delivery is not imminent

perfusion and aid in fetal resuscitation. In the case of severe variable decelerations or a sudden bradycardia during active labor or with rupture of membranes, an immediate cervical examination for possible cord prolapse should be performed. If no cord is palpated and variable decelerations continue, amnioinfusion (infusion of isotonic saline through an intrauterine catheter) should be considered to alleviate cord compression. Oxygen at 4 L/min should be administered to the mother to improve fetal oxygenation in all cases of suspected distress. Finally, if signs of distress are ongoing and delivery is not imminent, a fetal scalp pH should be performed to directly assess the fetal acid-base status.

Fetal scalp pH is the "gold standard" of antepartum assessment; scalp sampling is performed when the fetal acid-base status is in question due to an abnormal fetal heart rate. The fetus is accessed via the dilated cervix, and blood is obtained in a capillary tube from a small scalp incision. If the cervix is not dilated or the vertex is at a very high station, scalp sampling is not possible. A sample may be obtained from the buttocks of a breech fetus. A pH over 7.25 is reassuring, while a pH under 7.20 is an indication for immediate delivery. If the pH is intermediate or if the ominous heart rate pattern persists, the pH must be redetermined promptly (Table 5–5). The fetal response to vigorous scalp stimulation may be used as an alternative to scalp blood sampling. If there is an acceleration in the heart rate with stimulation (rubbing the scalp vigorously or puncturing as with blood sampling) a normal pH can be assumed. In the absence of acceleration with stimulation, the pH must be determined.

TABLE 5–5.
Measuring for an Abnormal Fetal Heart Rate

Maternal position change
Maternal oxygen therapy
Cervical examination and scalp stimulation
Discontinuation of oxytocin treatment
Consider amnioinfusion
Consider scalp pH

LIMITATIONS OF FETAL HEART RATE MONITORING

It is important to remember the limitations of fetal heart rate monitoring as a management tool in labor and delivery. False-negative results are uncommon, and a normal fetal heart rate is good evidence for a healthy fetus; exceptions are fetuses with some congenital anomalies. However, fetal heart rate monitoring is a less specific than sensitive tool, and false-positive results are common. A vigorous fetus is often surgically delivered after a diagnosis of fetal distress. This discrepancy can be due to decreased variability in fetal sleep states or to medications such as narcotics. Fetal recovery after an acute insult such as maternal hypotension is another cause of a false-positive test result. Interobserver variability in interpretation is substantial. As with most screening tests, the positive predictive value of fetal heart rate monitoring decreases with decreasing population risk. Thus, low-risk patients, who are less likely to benefit from continuous monitoring, are also more likely to suffer from unnecessary intervention due to erroneous testing or interpretation. A final problem with intrapartum heart rate monitoring is the difficulty of interpretation in premature labor patients, who form a substantial proportion of the high-risk population. Despite its limitations, however, fetal heart rate monitoring has become an important tool for intrapartum evaluation of high-risk pregnancies. Due to its ease of application and relative safety, continued use of this method is ensured until a practical and more accurate alternative becomes available.

ADDITIONAL READING

Leveno KJ, Cunningham FG: Forecasting fetal health, in Pritchard JA, MacDonald PC, Gant NF (eds): *Williams Obstetrics,* ed 17, suppl 19. E Norwalk, Conn, Appleton-Century-Crofts, 1988.

MacDonald D, Grant A, Sheridan-Pereira M, et al: The Dublin randomized controlled trial of intrapartum fetal heart rate monitoring. *Am J Obstet Gynecol* 1985; 152:524.

Prentice A, Lind T: Fetal heart rate monitoring during labour—too frequent intervention, too little benefit? Occasional survey. *Lancet* 1987; 331:1375.

Redman GWC: Fetal monitoring in labour. *BMJ* 1986; 292:6518.

MANAGEMENT OF DYSTOCIA 6

Dystocia, from the Greek *tokos,* or "birth," refers to abnormal progression of labor or childbirth. Dystocia can be due to a variety of factors; often these factors are characterized as "passage," "passenger," or "powers." Simply defined, the pelvis may be too small or misshaped, the fetus may be too large or anomalous, or the uterine contractions may be inadequate. Dystocia can occur at any point during labor; management depends on identifying the causative factor.

PHYSIOLOGY OF LABOR

A brief review of the physiology of labor will aid in understanding the mechanisms and treatment of dystocia. Uterine muscle differs from skeletal muscle in that myometrial cells are dispersed throughout a collagen matrix so that the muscle may pull in a variety of directions. The potential for shortening of myometrium is also much greater than in skeletal muscle. The muscle cells are integrated through gap junctions; gap junction formation is favored by increased prostaglandin levels and an increased estrogen/progesterone ratio. The number of gap junctions increases as pregnancy progresses (Fig 6–1).

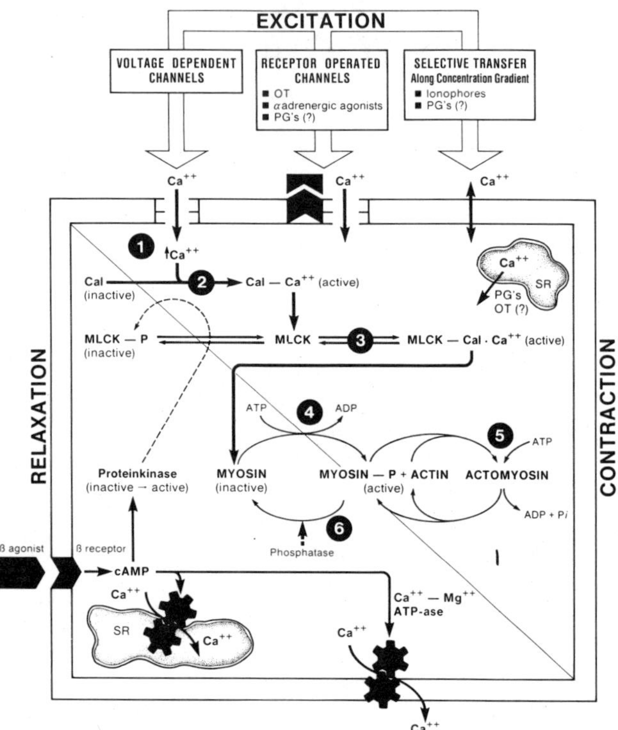

FIG 6–1.
Mechanism of uterine contraction. (*OT* = oxytocin; *PG* = prostaglandin; *SR* = sarcoplasmic retinaculum; *MLCK* = myosin light-chain kinase; *ATP* = adenosine triphosphate; *AMP* = adenosine monophosphate; *cAMP* = cyclic AMP.) (From Gabbe SG, Niebyl JR, Simpson JL: *Obstetrics*. New York, Churchill Livingstone, 1986. Used by permission.)

Myometrial contraction is effected when the protein filaments actin and myosin interact (slide past one another). Myosin contains a "head" region that has an actin-combining site, adenosine triphosphatase (ATPase), and "light chains." Phosphorylation of the myosin light chains by the calcium-activated enzyme myosin light-chain kinase (MLCK) is essential for muscle contraction; muscle relaxation occurs with the dephosphorylation of myosin by a phosphatase. MLCK can be inhibited by phosphorylation by a cyclic adenosine monophosphate (cAMP)-dependent kinase. cAMP also promotes calcium uptake. Calcium and cAMP are thus essential regulators of uterine muscle contraction; increased cAMP levels promote relaxation, while calcium promotes contraction. Hormonal regulation of myometrial activity involves these regulators; for example, prostaglandins and oxytocin inhibit calcium sequestration and increase myometrial activity (see Fig 6–1).

The physiologic mechanisms involved in initiation of labor in sheep are well described, but initiation of human parturition is still largely a mystery. Prostaglandins, known to stimulate uterine contraction, are produced both in decidua and amnion from arachidonic acid through calcium-dependent phospholipase action (Fig 6–2). Their exact role in initiating labor is still unknown; their levels increase in amniotic fluid and maternal plasma during but not before labor. Similarly, increased systemic estrogen and decreased progesterone, known to stimulate labor in other species, does not appear to be a trigger for labor in humans. However, fetal adrenal production of dehydroepiandrosterone sulfate, the precursor for placental production

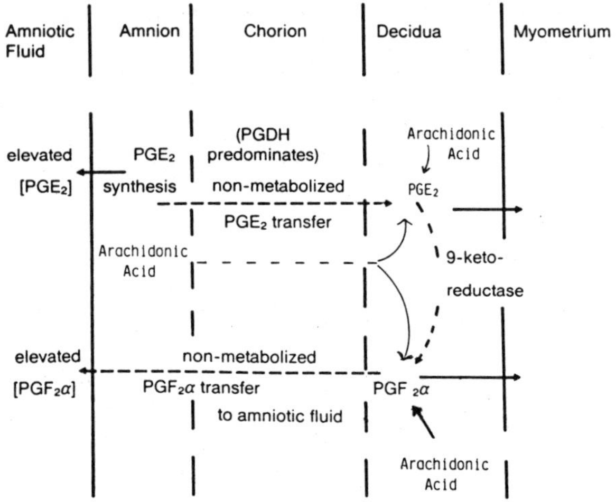

FIG 6–2.
Physiology of labor. (*PGE_2* = prostaglandin E_2; *PDGH* = 15-hydroxyprostaglandin dehydrogenase; *$PGF_{2\alpha}$* = prostaglandin $F_{2\alpha}$.)

of estradiol, appears to be necessary for labor because its absence delays labor onset. Finally, oxytocin, a potent uterine stimulant, increases in late pregnancy and during labor in maternal serum but does not increase acutely immediately prior to labor. Although systemic changes in prostaglandins, oxytocin, and steroid hormones have not been demonstrated, these compounds may still be involved in triggering labor through local changes in concentration.

For example, estrogen affects myometrium by increasing oxytocin receptors; increased local estrogen might increase the effect on myometrium of the stable oxytocin concentration. Research in this area is ongoing.

Although the exact mechanism of labor initiation is still under investigation, our current understanding has allowed the development of clinically useful tools to induce or augment labor. Prostaglandins can stimulate uterine contraction but are difficult to titrate; thus uterine hyperstimulation causing fetal distress is possible. Large doses of potent prostaglandins are thus generally used only for inducing abortion or for postpartum uterine atony. Smaller doses of less potent prostaglandin are used to promote cervical ripening but usually do not initiate active labor.

The mainstay of therapeutic induction or augmentation of labor is synthetic oxytocin. Oxytocin in an octapeptide similar to vasopressin and is generally given intravenously. Its half-life is 1 to 3 minutes, and it is cleared by liver, kidney, breast, and plasma oxytocinase. Aside from uterine and breast myoepithelial cell effects, oxytocin also has weak antidiuretic properties and can cause water intoxication. Large doses can also cause transient vasodilation with severe hypotension, particularly in the face of bleeding. Careful titration of the dose and fetal and uterine monitoring are essential since uterine hyperstimulation is possible.

LABOR DISORDERS

The normal first and second stages of labor have been described in Chapter 4. Dysfunctional labor can occur in the form of a prolonged latent phase, a protracted active phase, or arrest of labor. Dilation, descent, or both may be affected. Disorders can be detected by close attention to the labor curve.

A prolonged latent phase is usually diagnosed after 20 hours in primiparas or 14 hours in multiparas. The diagnosis may be confused by using the terms "true" and "false" labor. A patient who is tired and uncomfortable does not want to hear that her labor is "false." A better term is "early" labor. A prolonged latent phase may be treated in one of two ways: oxytocin augmentation with or without amniotomy or rest with sedation. Either therapy is effective in the majority of patients. Sedatives should be used only after exclusion of fetal distress or other indications for prompt delivery. The most common medication used in this situation is morphine, 15 mg intramuscularly.

A protracted active phase is diagnosed when the patient dilates at a rate less than 1 cm/hr, or 1.5 cm/hr in a multipara. Initiation of epidural anesthesia can decrease contractions for a short period of time (up to 30 minutes), and this should be considered when the diagnosis of a protracted active phase is made. This labor disorder may be caused by inadequate uterine contractions or cephalopelvic disproportion (30%) and is often associated with abnormal fetal head position (asynclitism). The first step in management is placement of an intrauterine pressure catheter to assess the adequacy of uterine contractions. If contractions are inadequate (less than three in 10 minutes or less than 50-mm pressure), oxytocin infusion is indicated; if contractions are adequate, the patient is observed for progress. If arrest of dilation occurs, cesarean section is indicated. It is important to note that even if labor progresses there is an increased risk of cephalopelvic disproportion. Assisted vaginal delivery in these patients increases the risk of birth injury.

Arrest disorders are characterized by a lack of dilation or descent over a period of 2 hours. Again, uterine contractions must be assessed and treated if inadequate. In the face of adequate contractions (50% of patients), treatment is cesarean section.

At times, the vertex will descend slowly to the +3 station with maternal pushing, but the second stage will be longer than the expected 2-hour maximum. The mother may be exhausted and require assisted delivery. It may be appropriate at this time to perform an episiotomy or apply outlet forceps or a vacuum device. In the absence of such a situation or other indications for immediate delivery, such measures are not recommended because they increase maternal trauma without demonstrable benefit to the fetus.

Cephalopelvic disproportion is frequently an indication for cesarean section. This should be considered in the management of a laboring patient with a history of cesarean section. Vaginal birth after cesarean (VBAC) is commonly recommended and has proved quite safe. However, in a patient with a history of true cephalopelvic disproportion, the chances for successful vaginal delivery at term are reduced by as much as 50%.

SHOULDER DYSTOCIA

Shoulder dystocia occurs in the course of vaginal delivery after the head is expelled (Fig 6–3). At this point, the shoulder normally rotates under the symphysis pubis and is delivered. In shoulder dystocia, the shoulder becomes lodged behind the symphysis, and the head retracts (the so-called turtle sign). Shoulder dystocia is an obstetric emergency. It is associated with an increased risk of fetal asphyxia or even death and with brachial plexus injury. Management consists of a series of maneuvers designed to dislodge the shoulder. McRobert's maneuver is attempted first. This entails further abduction and flexion of the mother's legs at the hips and increases the pelvic diameter by about 1 cm. Suprapubic (not fundal) pressure over the shoulder is applied next, along with pressure on the baby's back to rotate the shoulder. If these maneuvers fail, a fourth-degree episiotomy is performed, the posterior of the arm is delivered, and the baby is rotated to the transverse plane. Finally, deliberate fracture of the clavicle may be attempted. Replacement of the baby in the uterus after general anesthesia followed by cesarean section has been described.

Risk factors for shoulder dystocia include instrumented delivery after protracted labor, maternal obesity or diabetes,

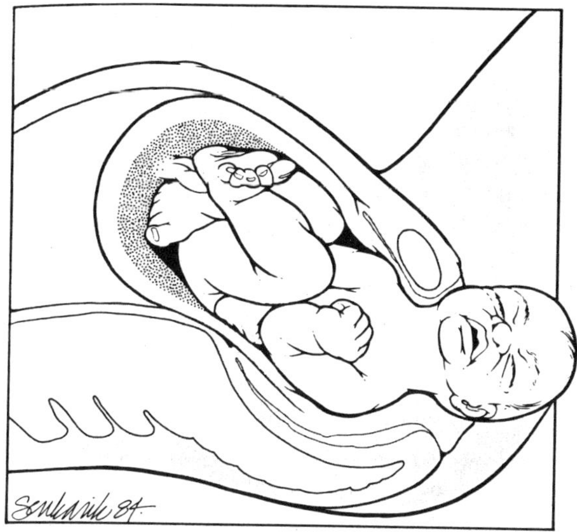

FIG 6–3.
Shoulder dystocia. (From Gabbe SG, Niebyl JR, Simpson JL: *Obstetrics*. New York, Churchill Livingstone, 1986. Used by permission.)

grand multiparity, and a large baby. Many shoulder dystocias occur in the absence of risk factors.

MALPRESENTATIONS

Dystocia may occur due to fetal malpresentation. Breech, transverse, compound, face, and brow presentations are uncommon at term but are frequently seen with premature labor. With a breech or transverse presentation, external cephalic version may be considered before the onset of active labor and rupture of the membranes. This is accomplished manually with the aid of a tocolytic agent such as terbutaline. Ultrasound and fetal heart rate monitoring are also used. The fetus is palpated through the maternal abdomen, and the buttocks are elevated. The head is held with the other hand, and slow, steady pressure is applied to reposition the fetus. Contraindications to version are fetal distress, prematurity, and anterior placenta or placental abruption, or decreased amniotic fluid (Table 6–1).

If version fails in a transverse lie, cesarean section is indicated. An actively laboring patient with the baby's shoulder presenting is in danger of rupturing her uterus.

A breech presentation may be managed with cesarean section or attempted vaginal delivery. For vaginal delivery, an experienced operator must be available. The estimated fetal size must be greater than 2500 g (with the exception

TABLE 6–1.
External Cephalic Version—Contraindications

Fetal distress
Prematurity
Anterior placenta
Placental abruption
Oligohydramios

of very low birth weight infants); smaller fetuses have a large head-abdomen ratio and are at risk for entrapment of the after-coming head. The fetus should be in a frank breech position with a flexed head, and the maternal pelvis should be evaluated and deemed adequate for the size of the fetus. If these criteria are met and labor progresses normally, vaginal breech delivery is quite safe.

Face and brow presentations are uncommon. In a face presentation, the chin (mentum) may be posterior, anterior, or transverse. Mentum anterior presentations are usually delivered vaginally, while mentum posterior or transverse presentations often require cesarean section. A face presentation is associated with an increased risk of fetal distress. A brow presentation may be manually corrected in some cases by elevation and flexion of the head. If this is unsuccessful, cesarean section is usually necessary.

A "compound presentation" refers to a hand or arm presenting with the vertex. Although this usually corrects itself during the course of labor, the risk of cord prolapse is increased, as in nonvertex presentations. The clinician should be aware of this possibility, and the fetus should be monitored. Cord prolapse is managed by elevation of the presenting part of the fetus to prevent cord compression while preparing for immediate cesarean section. Most compound presentations are delivered vaginally without intervention.

OBSTETRIC ANESTHESIA

The control of labor pain is an increasingly available option for the patient; it is also an essential clinical tool for the management of complicated labor. The use of narcotics in the latent phase and nonpharmacologic methods have already been mentioned. Other anesthetic options for childbirth include conduction and inhalation anesthesia. Narcotic use beyond the latent phase of labor is not recommended because the interval to birth may be short and neonatal clearance of narcotics is limited.

Conduction anesthesia includes local infiltration as for an episiotomy, pudendal block (injected through the vagina at the ischial spines) for delivery, paracervical block, subarachnoid block, and epidural block. A paracervical block is quite effective for control of pain from uterine contractions but is seldom used due to concern for fetal safety. A subarachnoid block (spinal) is often used for cesarean section. An epidural block is commonly used for labor and delivery. Lumbar epidural anesthesia can provide labor analgesia or surgical anesthesia depending on the types and doses of medication used. Caudal epidural anesthesia provides excellent pain control for the second stage of labor (Table 6–2).

Local anesthetics are generally used for regional anesthesia; increasingly, narcotic preparations for spinal and epidural injection are also being used. Unlike systemic narcotics, agents injected regionally or locally rarely enter the fetal compartment in significant quantity. Maternal side effects can include lidocaine (or other local anesthetic) tox-

TABLE 6–2.
Obstetric Anesthesia

Conduction anesthesia
Local infiltration
Pudendal block
Paracervical block (nonviable fetuses only)
Spinal block
Lumbar epidural block
Caudal epidural block
Inhalation anesthesia
Nitrous oxide
Rapid sequence
Narcotics (first stage only)

icity from inadvertent vascular injection or hypotension from sympathetic blockade with spinal or epidural anesthesia. The effect of epidural anesthesia on labor and delivery has been debated. It is clear that a temporary decrease in contractions can occur with initiation of epidural anesthesia, but other effects are more controversial. The rate of assisted delivery is increased in patients receiving epidural blocks, but this may be due to selection bias; patients with abnormal labor more often require anesthesia. Often initiation of anesthesia actually improves the labor pattern, presumably by decreasing anxiety and promoting relaxation.

Inhalation anesthesia is occasionally used in a laboring patient. Nitrous oxide is rapidly cleared and relatively safe for the fetus for short periods of time. It is less effective than epidural anesthesia but may be adequate in a patient experiencing a very rapid labor. Other inhalational agents are used mainly for induction of general anesthesia for cesarean section, although halothane is a potent uterine relaxant and can be used, for example, to aid in the management of an inverted uterus.

Studies show that emotional support throughout labor can have beneficial effects on the labor. Such support can decrease cesarean section rates, the need for anesthesia, and the length of labor.

SUMMARY

The goal of a clinician caring for a laboring patient is safe delivery of a healthy infant. To that end, careful monitoring and meticulous attention to labor progress and fetal well-being are essential. Knowledge of the patient's history, psychological state, physical condition, and labor risk factors will facilitate optimal care. Knowledge of pelvic architecture and fetal size, position, and presentation will take much of the guess workout of labor management. Above all, the great challenge of obstetrics is to actively and safely manage labor while supporting the patient in her desire for a happy and natural experience.

ADDITIONAL READING

Akoury HA, MacDonald FJ, Brodie G, et al: Oxytocin augmentation of labor and perinatal outcome in nulliparas. *Obstet Gynecol* 1991; 78:227.

Benedetti TJ, Lowensohn RI, Truscott AM: Face presentation at term. *Obstet Gynecol* 1980; 55:199.

Bingham P, Lilford RJ: Management of the selected term breech presentation: Assessment of the risks of selected vaginal delivery versus cesarean section for all cases. *Obstet Gynecol* 1987; 69:965.

Boylan PC: Labor in the primigravid patient. *Curr Probl Obstet Gynecol* 1991; 14:9.

Brindley BA, Sokol RJ: Induction and augmentation of labor: Basis and methods for current practice. *Obstet Gynecol Surv Rev* 1988; 43:730.

Carsten ME, Miller JD: A new look at uterine muscle contraction. *Am J Obstet Gynecol* 1987; 157:1303.

Casey ML, MacDonald PC: Biomolecular processes in the initiation of parturition: Decidual activation. *Clin Obstet Gynecol* 1988; 31:533.

Cetrulo CL: The controversy of mode of delivery in twins: The intrapartum management of twin gestation (Part I). *Semin Perinatol* 1986; 10:39.

Chervenak FA: The controversy of mode of delivery in twins: The intrapartum management of twin gestation (Part II). *Semin Perinatol* 1986; 10:44.

Ferguson JE, Armstrong MA, Dyson DC: Maternal and fetal factors affecting success of antepartum external cephalic version. *Obstet Gynecol* 1987; 70:722.

Hopwood HG Jr: Shoulder dystocia: Fifteen years' experience in a community hospital. *Am J Obstet Gynecol* 1982; 144:162.

Kennell J, Klaus M, McGrath SM, et al: Continuous emotional support during labor in a US hospital. *JAMA* 1991; 265:2197.

Lopez-Zeno JA, Peaceman AM, Adashek JA, et al: A controlled trial of a program for the active management of labor. *N Engl J Med* 1992; 326:450.

Modanlou H, Komatsu G, Dorchester W, et al: Large-for-gestational-age neonates: Anthropometric reasons for shoulder dystocia. *Obstet Gynecol* 1982; 60: 417.

Myers SA, Gleicher N: Breech delivery: Why the dilemma? *Am J Obstet Gynecol* 1986; 155:6.

Petrie RH: The pharmacology and use of oxytocin. *Clin Perinatol* 1981; 8:35.

Piper JM, Bolling DR, Newton ER: The second stage of labor: Factors influencing duration. *Am J Obstet Gynecol* 1991; 165:976.

Thorp JA, Boylan PC, Parisi VM, et al: Effects of high-dose oxytocin augmentation on umbilical cord blood gas values in primigravid women. *Am J Obstet Gynecol* 1988; 159:670.

Wallace D, Cunningham FG: Obstetrical anesthesia, in Pritchard JA, MacDonald PC, Gant NF (eds): *Williams Obstetrics,* ed 17, suppl 20. E Norwalk, Conn, Appleton-Century-Crofts, 1988.

COMPLICATED LABOR 7

Labor may be complicated by prematurity, premature rupture of membranes, vaginal bleeding, infection, breech delivery, delivery of twins, or preeclampsia. This is a brief overview of the most commonly encountered problems influencing labor management.

PREMATURITY

Prematurity is the leading cause of perinatal mortality in the developed world today. Premature labor is usually idiopathic, although some cases may be caused by infection, uterine anomalies, an incompetent cervix, or placental abnormalities. Despite extensive efforts to design an effective therapy for premature labor, little progress has been made in prolonging pregnancy once labor has begun. The major improvement in perinatal survival in such pregnancies has been the result of improvements in neonatal care.

Management of premature labor varies among practitioners. In the United States, tocolytic (contraction-inhibiting) therapy is popular. Medications commonly used are intravenous magnesium sulfate, parenteral β-sympathomimetics, antiprostaglandins, and calcium channel blockers. Each of these agents has a different and logical action in blocking the mechanism of labor. It is important to realize, however, that such therapies have to date been shown to have only limited usefulness. In placebo-controlled trials, these medications have been shown to prolong pregnancy for only short periods of time, on the order of days. This benefit must be weighed against the potential risks to the mother. Prolonged therapy with parenteral or oral tocolytics has not been shown to improve pregnancy outcome (Table 7–1).

Two new technologies have recently come into widespread use in the United States. These are home uterine activity monitoring and terbutaline pump therapy. The former is based on the theory that early detection and treatment of uterine contractions before labor becomes advanced may result in better success for tocolytic therapy. At-risk women monitor their uterine activity by using tocodynometry at home and transmit the results via phone lines. If frequent contractions are detected, therapy can be instituted immediately. Limited information is available on the success rate of such monitoring. Terbutaline pump therapy is even more poorly studied. This therapy involves continuous low-dose infusion of terbutaline, a β-sympathomimetic medication, with a device similar to the insulin pump. Despite its widespread use and very high cost, no study to date has demonstrated its safety or efficacy.

PREMATURE RUPTURE OF MEMBRANES

Another presentation for premature labor is premature rupture of membranes prior to labor. Such cases are managed

TABLE 7–1.

Tocolytic Therapy

Drug	Mechanism	Complications
Magnesium sulfate	? Calcium antagonist	Respiratory depressant in high doses
β-Mimetics	Increased cyclic adenosine monophosphate intracellularly	Myocardial ischemia, pulmonary edema, hyperglycemia
Nonsteroidal anti-inflammatory agents	Blocks prostaglandins	Decreased amniotic fluid, premature closure of ductus arteriosus
Calcium channel blockers	Blocks calcium influx	Reports of fetal death in animals

expectantly if the pregnancy has not reached the 36th week of gestation and no evidence of fetal distress or infection is seen. This approach is safe and of proven benefit to the fetus. Tocolytic or steroid therapy is not effective in these cases. Major risks with preterm premature rupture of membranes are infection and cord compromise; therefore, close maternal and fetal monitoring are warranted (Table 7–2).

Premature rupture of membranes may also occur at term. Considerable controversy exists as to whether expectant management or labor induction is the best mode of management. If the cervix is favorable (dilation >1 cm; effacement, >50%), labor induction after 12 to 24 hours is indicated. If the cervix is unfavorable, some practitioners opt to observe the patient until spontaneous labor begins in order to decrease the chances that cesarean delivery will be needed (see Table 7–2).

TABLE 7–2.

Management of Premature Rupture of Membranes

- Group B *Streptococcus* culture
- Minimal vaginal examination
- Preterm
  - Consider amniocentesis
  - Expectant management with fetal surveillance and bed rest
  - Monitor for signs of infection
- Term
  - Oxytocin (Pitocin) if no labor in 12 hr and favorable cervix
  - Expectant management 12–72 hr if unfavorable cervix

Delivery of a premature infant is conducted in much the same manner as a term delivery. If the fetus is vertex and has no evidence of fetal distress, cesarean delivery does not confer any advantage to the fetus. In the case of a breech presentation in an extremely premature fetus (<34 weeks), head entrapment is a danger, and cesarean delivery is recommended. Elective forceps in an attempt to protect the infant's head from birth trauma has not been shown to be effective. Conversely, most practitioners feel that a generous episiotomy may be protective.

VAGINAL BLEEDING

Bleeding at the time of labor may be due to a variety of etiologies. Many women have "bloody show," a consequence of normal cervical dilation. This is usually combined with cervical mucus and is seldom heavy. Painless heavy bleeding is the hallmark of placenta previa (Fig 7–1) or, less commonly, vasa previa. Either is an obstetric emergency, life-threatening to mother or baby. Bleeding accompanied by uterine tetany is the classic presentation for abruptio placentae. Again, immediate action is necessary to safeguard the mother and fetus.

The management of obstetric hemorrhage consists of obtaining maternal vital signs, establishing intravenous access, marshaling the delivery team, and assessing and maintaining hemodynamic stability with crystalloid and blood products. As soon as the maternal condition is deemed stable, fetal assessment and possibly delivery should be undertaken. In the case of vasa previa or pla-

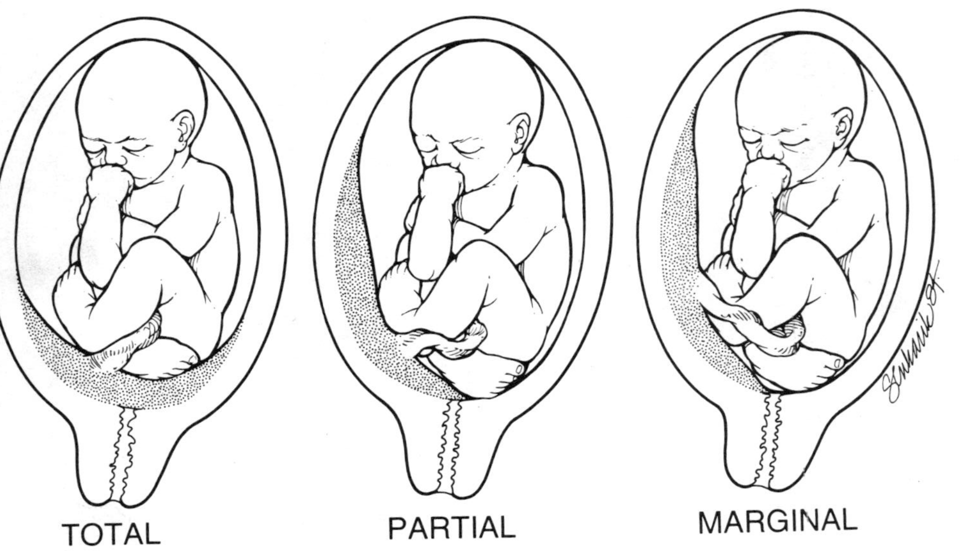

FIG 7–1.
Placenta previa. (From: Gabbe SG, Niebyl JR, Simpson JL. *Obstetrics*. New York, Churchill Livingstone, 1986. Used by permission.)

centa previa, this usually requires immediate cesarean delivery. In the case of placental abruption, the extent of abruption and condition of the mother and fetus will determine the mode of delivery.

Placental examination is important following delivery. Placental variations such as marginal insertion of the umbilical cord can be associated with fetal distress. Vasa previa or succenturiate lobes can also be seen on placental examination (Fig 7–2).

INFECTION

Infection can occur in conjunction with premature labor or premature rupture of membranes or may be a result of prolonged labor. Amnionitis as evidenced by fever, fetal or maternal tachycardia, uterine tenderness, or cloudy amniotic fluid should be treated with parenteral antibiotics. A standard regimen is ampicillin with or without gentamicin. The advantage of ampicillin is that it is known to penetrate the amniotic cavity. Furthermore, it is highly effective against group B *Streptococcus,* the most important pathogen in labor.

Amnionitis is not an indication for cesarean delivery. In fact, the risk to the mother of cesarean delivery is greatly increased in the face of infection. However, infection can cause uterine atony requiring oxytocin augmentation. Postpartum hemorrhage is also common for this reason. Following vaginal delivery it is uncommon for infection to persist. Conversely, postpartum endometritis is highly correlated with cesarean delivery in the face of amnionitis.

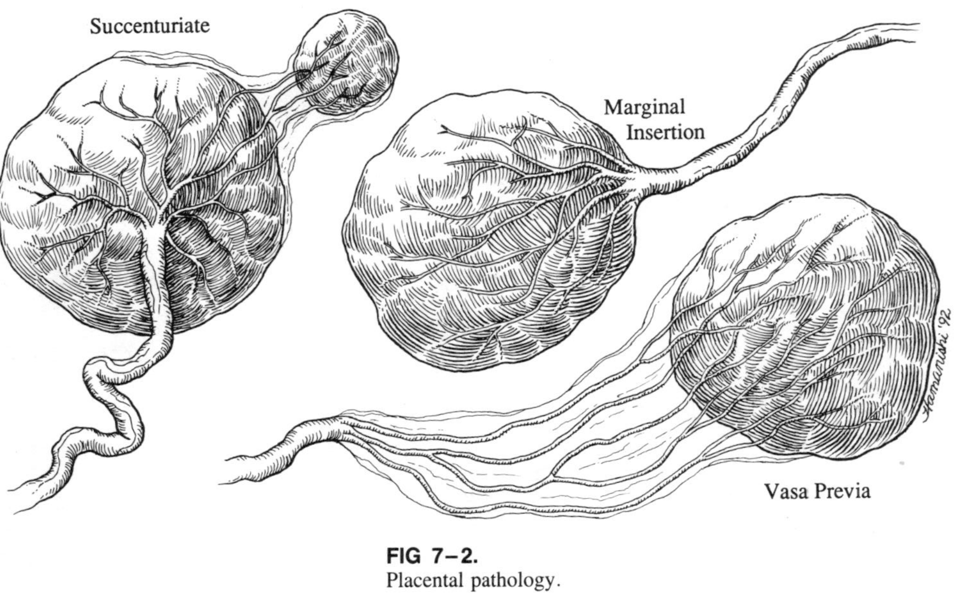

FIG 7–2.
Placental pathology.

BREECH DELIVERY

Considerable controversy surrounds the management of breech presentation; experienced obstetricians have varying opinions regarding the safety of vaginal delivery for the breech fetus. Part of the reason for this confusion is due to the association of breech presentation with fetal anomalies and with prematurity; these pregnancies would be expected to have worse outcomes regardless of the mode of delivery. However, a normal term or near-term fetus can be safely delivered by an experienced operator in the proper circumstances.

The desirable circumstance for a breech delivery includes gestational age greater than 34 weeks, fetal weight greater than 2500 g, a frank breech position with a flexed head, and a proven pelvis (previous vaginal delivery) or adequate pelvimetry. Labor should progress smoothly without evidence of fetal distress and preferably without a need for oxytocin augmentation. At the time of delivery, anesthesia should be available and the capability for cesarean delivery at hand. Informed consent from the patient regarding the risk of head entrapment must be obtained.

The mechanism of a breech delivery can be discussed in terms similar to that of a vertex delivery. *Engagement* occurs when the fetal bitrochanteric diameter enters the pelvic inlet. The point of reference is the fetal sacrum instead of the occiput. *Internal rotation* involves the bitrochanteric diameter rotating to the anteroposterior diameter of the pelvis. With *descent,* the bitrochanteric diameter passes under the symphysis and emerges transverse to the sacrum. *Rotation* occurs anterior to the sacrum, and the umbilicus appears. To this point the operator should have minimal involvement in the delivery; active traction can cause a startle reflex in the baby and predispose to nuchal arms, thereby complicating delivery. When the fetus is delivered up to the umbilicus, the thighs should be externally rotated to deliver the legs. As the scapula appears, the arms should be swept across the chest and delivered. At this point the baby is supported at the level of the perineum, and care must be taken to not hyperextend the neck. Suprapubic pressure is applied, and the head is flexed for delivery. Delivery of the head may be assisted by Piper forceps.

DELIVERY OF TWINS

Twin delivery is dependent on many factors, with fetal presentation being the most important. Twin pregnancies have a higher risk for a number of obstetric complications, including prematurity, hypertension, growth retardation, and fetal and placental anomalies. Any one of these may be overriding at the time of delivery. However, in an otherwise uncomplicated twin pregnancy with vertex-presenting twins, vaginal delivery is the mode of choice. A nonvertex-presenting twin is usually an indication for cesarean delivery (Table 7–3).

The first stage of labor in a twin delivery is conducted much as a singleton birth. Both twins should be carefully monitored. In the second stage following delivery of the

TABLE 7–3.
Delivery of Twins

Presentation	Second Twin	Method
Vertex	Nonvertex	Vaginal
Vertex	Vertex	Vaginal
Nonvertex	Nonvertex	Cesarean section
Nonvertex	Vertex	Cesarean section

first twin, placental integrity and position and the condition of the second fetus must be assessed. Delivery should be conducted in a setting where anesthesia is available and the capability for doing an immediate cesarean delivery exists. It is desirable to have a real-time ultrasound machine in the room to assess fetal position. In addition, oxytocin (Pitocin) and a uterine relaxant should be at hand. Pediatric support is desirable. After the first baby is delivered, the cord is clamped and cut, and the position of the second fetus is determined with ultrasound and manual examination. Fetal heart rate monitoring is continued. There is some risk at this point of premature separation of the placenta, and the patient must be watched closely for bleeding. In addition, Pitocin augmentation is often needed because there may be a lull in uterine contractions. If the second twin is vertex, descent of the head usually occurs rapidly, and the practitioner may guide the head into the pelvis or simply wait. Rupture of membranes should not be performed until the head is engaged to prevent cord prolapse. Delivery of the vertex second twin then proceeds as for a singleton. If the second twin is nonvertex, breech extraction is indicated. Through intact membranes, a foot or feet are firmly grasped, and gentle traction is applied. When the legs and body have been delivered up to the scapula, delivery proceeds as for a singleton breech presentation. Due to the need for manipulation, anesthesia in the form of a lumbar epidural block is usually recommended prior to the second stage. Numerous recent studies have shown that vaginal delivery in the face of a vertex-presenting twin and a nonvertex second twin of similar or smaller size is safe for both fetuses. No data are available on vaginal birth for higher-order gestations (triplets, etc.), and these patients are usually delivered by cesarean section.

PREECLAMPSIA

Preeclampsia (pregnancy-induced hypertension) complicates approximately 7% of pregnancies. This disease can be recognized by elevation of blood pressure by 30 points systolic or 15 points diastolic over first trimester values or by persistent blood pressures greater than 140/90. The elevated blood pressure is accompanied by edema and proteinuria. The etiology of preeclampsia is unknown. It is more frequently encountered in very young or older gravidas; in those with preexisting hypertension, renal disease, or other vascular disease; and in those with previous or a family history of preeclampsia. It is more common in first pregnancies. Patients with preeclampsia develop renal compromise in the form of nephropathy and renal insufficiency, coagulation abnormalities including thrombocytopenia, and hepatic abnormalities reflected by elevated transaminase levels.

HELLP syndrome (**h**emolysis, **e**levated **l**iver **e**nzymes, **l**ow **p**latelets) occurs in a subset of preeclamptics. Untreated preeclamptics may develop eclampsia (seizures), hepatic subcapsular hematomas, or disseminated intravascular coagulation. The fetus is also directly at risk since these patients are prone to abruptio placentae and uteroplacental insufficiency.

The cure for preeclampsia is delivery. In cases remote from term, expectant management or antihypertensive therapy may be attempted with close observation. In either case, treatment with parenteral magnesium sulfate to prevent seizures is indicated, particularly during labor and for 24 hours postpartum. Other antiseizure medications are sometimes used, but magnesium sulfate is the current U.S. standard of care. Delivery of preeclamptics may be vaginally or by cesarean section, depending on the condition of the mother and fetus. In the case of eclampsia, as with hemorrhage, the maternal condition must be stabilized prior to any attempt at delivery.

ADDITIONAL READING

Abdella TN, Siba BM, Hays JM, et al: Relationship of hypertensive disease to abruptio placentae. *Obstet Gynecol* 1984; 63:365.

Benedetti TJ: Maternal complications of parenteral β-sympathomimetic therapy for premature labor. Clinical opinion. *Am J Obstet Gynecol* 1983; 145:1.

Besinger RE, Niebyl JR: The safety and efficacy of tocolytic agents for the treatment of preterm labor. *Obstet Gynecol Surv* 1990; 45:415.

Boyer DM, Gotoff SP: Prevention of early-onset neonatal group B streptococcal disease with selective intrapartum chemoprophylaxis. *N Engl J Med* 1986; 314:1665.

Conway, DI, Prendiville WJ, Morris A, et al: Management of spontaneous rupture of the membranes in the absence of labor in primigravid women at term. *Am J Obstet Gynecol* 1984; 150:947.

Cox SM, Williams ML, Leveno KJ: The natural history of preterm ruptured membranes: What to expect of expectant management. *Obstet Gynecol* 1988; 71:558.

Dudley DK, Hardie MJ: Fetal and neonatal effects of indomethacin used as a tocolytic agent. *Am J Obstet Gynecol* 1985; 151:181.

Duff P, Huff RW, Gibbs RS: Management of premature rupture of membranes and unfavorable cervix in term pregnancy. *Obstet Gynecol* 1984; 63:697.

Garite TJ. Premature rupture of the membranes: The enigma of the obstetrician. Clinical opinion. *Am J Obstet Gynecol* 1985; 151:1001.

Gray BM, Egan ML, Pritchard DG: The group B streptococci: From natural history to the specificity of antibodies. *Semin Perinatol* 1990; 14(suppl 1):10.

Harris BA Jr: Peripheral placental separation: A review. *Obstet Gynecol Surv* 1988; 43:577.

King JF, Grant A, Keirse M, et al: Beta-mimetics in preterm labour: An overview of the randomized controlled trials. *Br J Obstet Gynaecol* 1988; 95:211.

Lowe TW, Cunningham FG: Placental abruption. *Clin Obstet Gynecol* 1990; 33:406.

Minkoff H, Mead P: An obstetric approach to the prevention of early-onset group B β-hemolytic streptococcal sepsis. Clinical opinion. *Am J Obstet Gynecol* 1986; 154:973.

Roberts JM, Taylor RN, Musci TJ, et al: Preeclampsia: An endothelial cell disorder. *Am J Obstet Gynecol* 1989; 161:1200.

Saftlas AF, Olson DR, Franks AL, et al: Epidemiology of preeclampsia and eclampsia in the United States, 1979–1986. *Am J Obstet Gynecol* 1990; 163:460.

Sibai BM, McCubbin JH, Anderson GD, et al: Eclampsia. I. Observations from 67 recent cases. *Obstet Gynecol* 1981; 58:609.

Wagner MV, Chin VP, Peters CJ, et al: A comparison of early and delayed induction of labor with spontaneous rupture of membranes at term. *Obstet Gynecol* 1989; 74:93.

Watson KV, Moldow CF, Ogburn PL, et al: Magnesium sulfate: Rationale for its use in preeclampsia. *Proc Natl Acad Sci U S A* 1986; 83:1075.

CASE PROBLEMS 8

This chapter provides readers with an opportunity to gain practical experience through 11 "real-world" case problems. Each case details the patient's clinical manifestations and management scenario. Readers are then asked to choose from among several treatment options. The discussion section of each case confirms the most appropriate choice from among the treatment options and discusses the related course of therapy.

CASE PROBLEM 1

The patient is a 20-year-old nullipara primigravida (G1 P0) at term. Her past history and antepartum course were uneventful, and her pelvis was evaluated as gynecoid and adequate clinically. Her contractions began 6 hours prior to admission and were somewhat irregular in that they occurred every 10 to 20 minutes. During the hour prior to admission, the contractions occurred every 2 to 5 minutes and lasted for 20 to 30 seconds. On admission the patient's blood pressure was 110/60 mm Hg; pulse, 84 per minute; and temperature, 37° C. The fundus measured 38 cm above the pubic symphysis with fetal heart tones heard in the right lower quadrant at 144 beats per minute. The estimated fetal weight was 7 lb.

Vaginal examination revealed a cervix that was 50% effaced, posterior, and firm. It was 1 cm dilated, and the vertex was presenting at the −1 station. The membranes were intact. The admission hematocrit was 35%. Admission urine revealed negative glucose and negative protein. An external electronic fetal monitoring strip revealed a fetal heart rate averaging 144 beats per minute with good variability and minimum acceleration noted at the time of contractions. Contractions were noted to be mild, lasted approximately 20 seconds, and occurred irregularly every 2 to 5 minutes.

The patient was observed for 2 hours, during which time the contractions became farther apart, occurred every 10 to 20 minutes, and still lasted approximately 20 seconds.

There was no change in the cervix, the position of the presenting part, or the fetal monitoring strip.

On the basis of the above information, what is the most likely diagnosis?

1. Prolonged latent phase
2. Braxton Hicks contractions (false labor)
3. Midpelvic cephalopelvic disproportion
4. Cervical dystocia

Discussion

True labor implies a progressive softening and dilatation of the cervix and descent of the head in the face of meaningful contractions. Generally, the contractions of true labor last in excess of 1 minute and come at regular intervals. During the latent phase, contractions generally become progressively stronger and more closely spaced, and the cervix effaces and dilates to approximately 3 cm. During this time the presenting part often descends into the pelvis and allows engagement to take place.

This patient has continued to have very mild, irregular contractions that are now becoming farther apart. There has been no evidence for continued descent or ripening or dilatation of the cervix. Therefore, a prolonged latent phase is less likely to be the diagnosis, and Braxton Hicks contractions (false labor) are the most likely condition. Although the vertex is near the ischial spines, there is probably not enough evidence to demonstrate midpelvic cephalopelvic disproportion at this stage of labor. Since the cervix has not ripened or dilated progressively, a cervical dysfunction problem is unlikely. In fact, one could question whether or not such a condition really exists.

Given the fact that the fetus appears to be in good condition, the best course of management for this patient would be discharge from the labor suite with mild sedation.

CASE PROBLEM 2

The patient is a 22-year-old G1 P0 at term. Her past history and antepartum course were uneventful, and her pelvis was deemed gynecoid and adequate clinically. Her contractions began 5 hours prior to admission and were somewhat irregular in that they occurred every 7 to 10 minutes. During the hour prior to admission the patient had been contracting every 5 minutes, and the contractions have lasted between 45 seconds and 1 minute. On admission to the hospital, the patient appeared quite uncomfortable during a contraction. Her blood pressure was 120/80 mm Hg; pulse, 92 per minute; and temperature, 37.1° C. The fundal height was 37 cm, and the estimated fetal weight was 7½ lb. Vaginal examination revealed the cervix to be 2 cm dilated, 50% effaced, and quite firm; the membranes were intact; and the presenting part was felt to be vertex at station 0. The fetal heart rate was noted at 136 beats per minute in the left lower quadrant. On admission her hematocrit was 36%, her urine was negative for protein and glucose, and a fetal monitoring strip revealed a fetal heart rate of 136 beats per minute on average with good variability and minimum accelerations during contractions.

Contractions continued at moderate intensity every 5 minutes and lasted approximately 1 minute. After 2 hours the cervical dilatation was thought to be 2 to 3 cm, and the cervix was approximately 70% effaced. The vertex remained at station 0 with the membranes intact. After 2 additional hours contractions continued at about the same interval and strength, but the patient was becoming quite tired and complained that the contractions were quite painful. Cervical examination revealed the cervix to still be 2 to 3 cm dilated and approximately 70% effaced, and the vertex continued at station 0 with the membranes intact. The fetal condition continued as priorly noted.

What is the most likely diagnostic possibility?

1. Prolonged latent stage
2. Braxton Hicks contractions (false labor)
3. Midpelvic cephalopelvic disproportion
4. Cervical dystocia

Discussion

This patient has had regular moderate, painful contractions with minimum cervical progress of effacement and dilatation over a 4-hour period. It is therefore unlikely that she is in false labor and more likely that she is demonstrating a prolonged latent phase. Progress in labor has not proceeded far enough to determine a cephalopelvic disproportion at the midpelvis, and as noted in the previous case, cervical dystocia is a difficult diagnosis to make or understand.

This patient would best be managed by amniotomy with the placement of a scalp electrode and internal pressure catheter followed by oxytocin augmentation in an attempt to shorten the prolonged latent phase. Oxytocin will help ripen the cervix and create a more meaningful labor pattern. One would then expect further dilatation of the cervix and descent of the vertex as the strength of the contractions is improved and their interval shortened. Mild sedation or an epidural anesthetic might also help at this point.

CASE PROBLEM 3

The patient is a 21-year-old G1 P0 at 41 weeks' gestation who noted the spontaneous rupture of her membranes 6 hours prior to admission. Within an hour of this, contractions began and have occurred every 4 to 6 minutes for the 6-hour period prior to admission. On admission the cervix is noted to be completely effaced and 4 cm dilated. The vertex is at the −2 station and left occipitoposterior (LOP) in position. The estimated fetal weight is 6½ lb. The patient's pelvis had previously been clinically typed as anthropoid, probably adequate for an average-sized baby, and this is once again the impression of the physician doing the assessment. The fundus is 36 cm above the pubic symphysis. The fetal heart rate is 144 beats per minute in the left lower quadrant. The fetal monitoring strip reveals a heart rate of approximately 144 beats per minute with good variability and accelerations with examination and contractions. The patient's vital signs, hematocrit, and urinalysis were all within normal limits.

At the time of the vaginal examination a copious amount of amniotic fluid was noted coming from the cervix, and an internal electrode was placed and an internal pressure catheter positioned. After 2 hours, her contractions were still noted to be every 4 to 6 minutes lasted approximately 1 minute, and were about 35 mm Hg in strength. The vertex is 5 cm in dilatation and 100% effaced, and the vertex is at station −1.

Two hours later the contractions are every 5 minutes and of about the same intensity. The cervix is still 5 cm dilated and completely effaced; the vertex is at −1, still LOP. The fetal heart tracings remain appropriately active.

Which of the following is the most likely circumstance?

1. Midpelvic arrest
2. Prolonged latent phase
3. Cephalopelvic disproportion.

Discussion

This patient most likely has an arrest at the midpelvis. This is not unusual in a narrow pelvis with prominent ischial spines, a presentation frequently seen in the anthropoid configuration. The vertex is in the LOP position, which indicates that the head is not well flexed. The station is still −1, which speaks against total engagement of the vertex into the pelvis.

From the time the patient entered into labor, the cervix has been effaced and greater than 4 cm dilated, so the latent phase has passed, and the patient must be considered to be in the active accelerated phase of labor. It is not possible to make the diagnosis of cephalopelvic disproportion since the patient has not had an adequate labor pattern and the circumstances noted above may be correctable.

Under the circumstances of this case, oxytocin should be begun with the goal of improving the strength of contractions to between 50 and 100 mm Hg and decreasing the interval of contraction to approximately 2 to 3 minutes. With an improvement in the force of labor, it is possible that the positional effect of the fetal head and narrow pelvis can be negotiated. Once good contractions have been established, if progress is not made within 2 hours, the patient is said to have had an adequate trial of labor, and cesarean delivery is indicated. However, if progress is made, the physician should show patience and allow the patient to progress until she either delivers or demonstrates a second arrest of progression.

CASE PROBLEM 4

The patient is a 24-year-old G3 P0 SAB(spontaneous abortion)1 TOP(termination of pregnancy)1 female at term who was admitted with a history of having had ruptured membranes 4 hours prior to admission and the onset of labor 3 hours prior to admission, and on admission she is found to be having contractions every 5 to 8 minutes that last 45 seconds and are of moderate quality to palpation. The patient's antepartum course has been benign. Her pelvis has been typed as android in configuration with a narrow pubic arch, converging sidewalls, a forward sacrum, and a narrow intraspinous diameter. The estimated fetal weight is 6 lb. The fetus is presenting in a right occipitoposterior (ROP) vertex presentation at the −2 station. The cervix is 5 cm dilated and 90% effaced. The fetal heart rate tracing shows a fetal heart rate that averages 140 beats per minute and has good variability. The patient's vital signs, admitting hematocrit, and urinalysis are all within the normal range.

After 2 hours the cervical dilatation and position of the vertex are unchanged, and the contractions are now every 8 to 10 minutes and mild to moderate. The fetal condition is stable as noted by monitoring (a scalp electrode was placed at the time of admission). A pressure catheter is inserted into the uterus, and the contractions are noted to be 30 to 40 mm Hg in strength. Because of this, oxytocin therapy is begun, and contractions improve in strength and interval. After 2 further hours, the contractions are occurring every 2 to 3 minutes, last 1 minute, and have a strength of 60 to 70 mm Hg. The cervix is now 8 cm dilated, but the vertex is still at the −2 station, and a good deal of molding is noted. The position is still ROP.

Which of the following is the best management plan for this patient's situation?

1. Continue oxytocin.
2. Perform a cesarean delivery.
3. Attempt to manually rotate the vertex and allow labor to continue.

Discussion

The vertex is still unengaged even though labor has improved. The patient is known to have an android pelvis and a posterior presentation of the vertex. The chances of vaginal delivery are small; however, the patient has continued to make progress with cervical dilatation, and there is no harm in continuing the oxytocin stimulation for a longer period of time. However, if the vertex does not descend within the next 1 to 2 hours, cephalopelvic disproportion can be assumed, and a cesarean delivery is appropriate. With the vertex at the −2 station, fetal molding apparent, and the cervix not fully dilated, an attempt at manual rotation would not be indicated. This maneuver should be utilized when the cervix is fully dilated, the vertex well engaged in the pelvis, and the pelvis deemed to be adequate for the fetal size.

CASE PROBLEM 5

The patient is a 39-year-old G5 P4 female at term. She enters with a history of having begun to note painful contractions every 5 to 10 minutes 4 hours prior to admission. Her membranes are intact. She had previously been typed as having a clinically gynecoid but small pelvis. All of her previous deliveries were vaginal, and all children are living and healthy. Her first pregnancy occurred 10 years ago, and a 3200-g fetus was delivered with midforceps at 40 weeks after 24 hours of labor. Her second pregnancy occurred 8 years ago and continued until 41 weeks of gestation. After an 18-hour labor, she was delivered of a 3000-g infant by low forceps. Her third pregnancy occurred 6 years ago, and she delivered a 2400-g infant spontaneously at 35 weeks' gestation after a 6-hour labor. Her fourth pregnancy occurred 2 years ago, and she delivered a 3100-g infant at 40 weeks' gestation after a 20-hour labor by low forceps.

Her antepartum course has been uneventful, and amniocentesis performed at 16 weeks' gestation revealed an infant with a 46, XX karyotype. On admission, the cervix is 90% effaced and 4 cm dilated, and the vertex is ballotable over the inlet and is floating. The membranes are bulging. The fundal height is 40 cm, and the estimated fetal weight is 8 lb. The fetal heart is heard at 140 beats per minute in the right lower quadrant. Her hematocrit is 32%, and a urine sample is negative for glucose and protein. Blood pressure is 110/70 mm Hg, and pulse, 88 per minute; and temperature, 37° C.

A fetal monitoring strip reveals a fetus with good beat-to-beat variability and mild acceleration with contractions. After 2 hours, the cervix is at 6-cm dilatation and 90% effaced, and the vertex is still floating at the inlet. At this point the contractions are occurring every 2 to 3 minutes and are moderate to strong. Shortly thereafter the membranes ruptured spontaneously. Examination reveals the vertex to be well approximated to a cervix that is 7 cm but is still at the −3 station. There is no evidence of a prolapsed umbilical cord, and the fetal heart rate tracing remains stable and reassuring. A scalp electrode is placed and an internal pressure catheter inserted.

Over the next 2 hours the contractions continue to be strong, last 1 minute, and occur every 2 to 3 minutes with a strength of 50 to 60 mm Hg. The patient is noted to be fully dilated. The vertex, however, remains at the −3 station. The patient is asked to bear down with contractions, which she does well. But after 1 hour and 45 minutes, the vertex has not descended any farther. The vertex is in the left occipitotransverse (LOT) presentation, and the examiner notes that some fairly significant caput is being raised. The fetal heart rate tracing remains stable.

At this point, which of the following should the obstetrician do?

1. Begin oxytocin.
2. Continue observation with bearing-down efforts on the part of the patient.
3. Do a cesarean delivery.

Discussion

The patient has been having good labor and has been bearing down adequately. In spite of this, the vertex remains high even though the patient has been in the second stage for an hour and 45 minutes. The fact that a caput is beginning to form demonstrates the likelihood that the fetus is not negotiating the birth canal. Oxytocin will probably not improve the already efficient contractions, and continuation of labor with bearing-down efforts will probably not help engage the head. The fact that the fetus is in the LOT position is not unusual for an unengaged vertex. This individual probably has an inlet cephalopelvic disproportion even though she has had four previous babies, some of whom have been fairly large; she does not seem able to deliver this baby vaginally. A cesarean delivery is an appropriate choice of management. Continuing labor has the risk of a ruptured uterus in a grand multiparous patient such as this or the development of a Bandl contraction ring and the development of fetal distress.

CASE PROBLEM 6

A 33-year-old G1 P0 at 41 weeks' gestation is admitted with labor pains and bloody show. Her pregnancy has been uncomplicated. She reports that she has had contractions for 3 hours and for the past 6 hours has had decreased fetal movement. On examination, the patient is normotensive and in moderate distress. Her cervix is 3 cm dilated and completely effaced; the vertex is at the −1 station. The patient requests and receives morphine for pain, and 2 hours later a lumbar epidural block is placed.

A review of the patient's external fetal heart rate tracing reveals an initial rate of 130 beats per minute with good variability and accelerations. Decreased variability is noted after the morphine, and the accelerations disappear. While the patient is on her side for epidural placement and injection, a marked fetal bradycardia occurs. Following the next two contractions, late decelerations are evident.

What is appropriate for evaluating the fetal heart rate and making a management plan?

1. Perform an immediate cesarean delivery.
2. Check the blood pressure and cervical dilation, and place a fetal scalp electrode.
3. Start oxygen therapy, change the maternal position, and observe.
4. Start an amnioinfusion.

Discussion

This patient had an apparently healthy fetus prior to placement of the epidural block. Because hypotension secondary to sympathectomy is common with epidural anesthesia, it is likely that temporary uterine hypoperfusion is causing the apparent fetal distress. The blood pressure should be measured and treated with ephedrine if low. It would be prudent to check cervical dilation, rupture the membranes to check for meconium, begin O_2 treatment, and place a fetal scalp electrode as well.

CASE PROBLEM 7

A 26-year-old G2 P0 presents at 36 weeks' gestation with a headache. Her history is remarkable for vaginal bleeding 2 days prior to admission. Currently she complains of menstrual-type cramping. On examination, her blood pressure is 160/110 mm Hg. Head and neck, cardiac, and pulmonary examinations are negative. Reflexes are 3+, and there is 2+ peripheral edema present. The cervix is 1 cm dilated. Laboratory findings include a creatinine value of 1.1 mg/dL, platelets of 141,000/dL, and a uric acid of 7.2 units. Her urine shows 2+ protein. External fetal monitors are placed. Fetal heart tones are 150 beats per minute with decreased variability; uterine irritability is seen. Magnesium sulfate infusion is begun, her membranes are ruptured, a fetal scalp electrode is placed, and oxytocin (Pitocin) induction of labor is begun.

Two hours later, her blood pressure remains 160/105. Contractions are every 3 minutes. Fetal heart tones are 160 beats per minute and nonreactive. On close examination of the fetal heart rate tracing, shallow decelerations are seen following each contraction. Cervical examination is unchanged except that meconium-stained amniotic fluid is now present. You are consulted and recommend which of the following?

1. Immediate cesarean delivery.
2. Perform a scalp pH.
3. Observe for 1 hour to see whether labor progresses.
4. Start an amnioinfusion.

Discussion

This patient has severe preeclampsia. It is also apparent that there is poor placental function and resultant fetal distress. In order to prevent fetal damage, immediate cesarean delivery is indicated.

CASE PROBLEM 8

An 18-year-old G2 P1 presents at 40 weeks with ruptured membranes. She has had an uncomplicated pregnancy, and the fluid is clear. On examination, her blood pressure is normal. The cervix is 3 cm and completely effaced, with the vertex at the 0 station. The patient is contracting every 3 minutes, and fetal heart tones are reactive by external monitoring.

Over the next 3 hours the patient feels increased pelvic pressure. Fetal heart tones continue to show good variability but also show moderate to severe variable decelerations with each contraction. On examination, the cervix is 6 cm dilated with the vertex at the +1 station. The fetal heart tones accelerate with the stimulation of the examination. Position change and oxygen therapy fail to alleviate the decelerations. What should be recommended?

1. Immediate cesarean delivery
2. Observation since the patient is making good progress in labor
3. Scalp pH
4. Amnioinfusion

Discussion

The patient has a healthy fetus. However, probably due to cord compression, repetitive variable decelerations persist. Because scalp stimulation results in fetal heart rate acceleration, a scalp pH is unnecessary. However, this patient may well benefit from amnioinfusion.

CASE PROBLEM 9

The patient is a 27-year-old G2 P1 female at 39 weeks' gestation who is admitted with a history of having begun labor 4 hours prior to admission; upon admission the contractions are found to be every 2 to 3 minutes and last about 1 minute. On examination the patient is noted to have a fundus of 38 cm, and the vertex is found in the right upper quadrant. The fetal heart rate is strong at 128 in the periumbilical area. A fetal monitoring strip reveals a fetal heart rate averaging 128 beats a minute with good variability. On vaginal examination, the membranes are found to be intact. The fetus is presenting in a frank breech position at station 0 with the cervix 4 cm dilated. The patient's pelvis is clinically typed as gynecoid and average to large.

The patient gives a previous history of having delivered an 8-lb baby spontaneously after an 8-hour labor. The estimated weight of the fetus is 7½ lb. Ultrasound examination reveals no obvious pelvic abnormalities and a head that is well flexed. The fetus appears to be without congenital malformations.

Which of the following is the best plan of management for this patient?

1. Cesarean delivery.
2. Allow labor and perform an assisted breech delivery.

3. Allow full dilatation and deliver by breech extraction.
4. Perform an external version.

Discussion

Several physicians in this era would perform a cesarean delivery on all breech presentations. However, there are no data to support that this means of delivery is superior to a vaginal breech delivery if the fetus is in the frank breech position in an adequate pelvis and the head is well flexed and is of a size that would be expected to be deliverable in a pelvis of this size and shape. In the current case, the buttocks are presenting, the fetus is of a weight comparable to the previous vertex delivery, the pelvis is adequate clinically, and the head is well flexed as noted by ultrasound. The breech is engaged since the presenting part is at station 0. Therefore, this would be the ideal patient to attempt a vaginal breech delivery. The patient, of course, must be well counseled as to the various risks and benefits of a vaginal breech vs. a cesarean delivery, and it is assumed that the operator has sufficient experience and skill to deliver a breech birth vaginally.

The safest course in vaginal breech delivery is to allow an assisted breech delivery, that is, to allow the breech to be delivered up to the umbilicus, disengage the legs, and then proceed with the completion of the delivery by using either Piper forceps on the after-coming head or the Mauriceau-Smellie-Veit maneuver. If there is no fetal distress, a breech extraction is usually not necessary and may increase the risk of damaging the fetus.

Although external versions are useful and may reduce the number of breech presentations, with labor already commenced and the breech engaged, the success rate would be low. A choice of whether or not to try a version and whether or not to use a tocolytic agent to relax the uterus would be left to the discretion of the operator. However, most obstetricians would not attempt a version at this stage of labor.

CASE PROBLEM 10

A 28-year-old G4 P2 is admitted at 33 weeks after the onset of regular strong contractions. Her pregnancy has been complicated only by first-trimester bleeding. She has had bloody show but no loss of fluid. The maternal examination is unremarkable, and the fetal heart tones are reactive. However, on abdominal examination, the fetus is felt to be breech. Vaginal examination shows the cervix to be 3 cm with small parts palpable.

You are asked to recommend therapy, but as you enter the room, spontaneous rupture of the membranes occurs. Immediate cervical examination reveals a 4-cm cervix with a foot palpable. Fetal heart tones now show mild variable decelerations. What should you recommend?

1. Close observation of fetal heart tones as labor progresses with frequent examinations of the cervix
2. Amnioinfusion
3. Cesarean delivery
4. Tocolytic therapy

Discussion

The patient has advanced labor with ruptured membranes at a viable gestational age. Tocolytic therapy is not indicated. Immediate cesarean delivery to avoid cord prolapse is the therapy of choice.

CASE PROBLEM 11

A 23-year-old G1 P0 with a 35-week twin gestation presents with contractions and bloody show. Both babies are appropriately grown, and the patient has had no other complications. On admission, the patient is normotensive and in mild distress. Her cervix is 5 cm dilated and completely effaced with the vertex of twin A at the 1+ station. Real-time ultrasound shows twin B to be in a frank breech position with a flexed head. What mode of delivery should be recommended for this patient?

1. Immediate cesarean delivery
2. Vaginal delivery of twin A followed by external version of twin B with vaginal delivery
3. Vaginal delivery of twin A and cesarean delivery for twin B
4. Vaginal delivery of both twins

Discussion

The mode of delivery in twins is controversial. However, there is good evidence that vaginal delivery of a breech second twin is safe. External version of the second twin does not confer an advantage to the fetus. Therefore, vaginal delivery is indicated with breech extraction of the second twin.

NOTES

NOTES

NOTES

NOTES

NOTES

INDEX